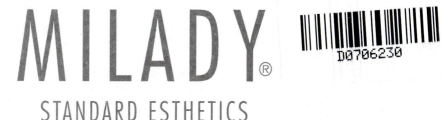

WORKBOOK

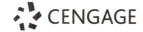

CENGAGE

Australia • Brazil • Mexico • Singapore • United Kingdom • United States

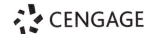

Milady Standard Esthetics: Fundamentals Workbook, 12th Edition

Milady

Vice President and General Manager, Milady: Sandra Bruce

Product Director: Kara Melillo

Product Manager: David Santillan

Learning Design Manager: Jessica Mahoney

Senior Content Manager: Nina Tucciarelli

Content Manager: Sarah Koumourdas

Learning Designer: Beth Williams

In-house Subject Matter Expert: Harry Garrott

Marketing Manager: Kim Berube

Marketing Director: Slavik Volinsky

Design Director, Creative Studio: Jack Pendleton

For product information and technology assistance, contact us at
Cengage Customer & Sales Support, 1-800-354-9706 or support.cengage.com.

For permission to use material from this text or product, submit all requests online at **www.cengage.com/permissions.**

Library of Congress Control Number: 2019938528

ISBN: 978-1-3370-9504-4

Cengage
20 Channel Center Street
Boston, MA 02210
USA

Cengage is a leading provider of customized learning solutions with employees residing in nearly 40 different countries and sales in more than 125 countries around the world. Find your local representative at: **www.cengage.com/global.**

Cengage products are represented in Canada by Nelson Education, Ltd.

For your lifelong learning solutions, visit www.milady.com

To register or access your online learning solution or purchase materials for your course, visit **www.cengage.com.**

Notice to the Reader

Publisher does not warrant or guarantee any of the products described herein or perform any independent analysis in connection with any of the product information contained herein. Publisher does not assume, and expressly disclaims, any obligation to obtain and include information other than that provided to it by the manufacturer. The reader is expressly warned to consider and adopt all safety precautions that might be indicated by the activities described herein and to avoid all potential hazards. By following the instructions contained herein, the reader willingly assumes all risks in connection with such instructions. The publisher makes no representations or warranties of any kind, including but not limited to, the warranties of fitness for particular purpose or merchantability, nor are any such representations implied with respect to the material set forth herein, and the publisher takes no responsibility with respect to such material. The publisher shall not be liable for any special, consequential, or exemplary damages resulting, in whole or part, from the readers' use of, or reliance upon, this material.

Printed in the United States of America
Print Number: 01   Print Year: 2019

CONTENTS

HOW TO USE THIS WORKBOOK

The *Milady Standard Esthetics: Fundamentals Workbook* has been especially designed to meet the needs, interests, and abilities of students receiving training for a career in esthetics, the art of skin care. It has been organized to be used in conjunction with *Milady Standard Esthetics: Fundamentals*, Twelfth Edition. Complete each workbook chapter as the textbook chapter is covered in class and you will be one step closer to preparing for your licensure exam and obtaining your license!

   This edition includes a wide variety of activities in order to engage you and to help you retain the information in each chapter. This workbook contains fill-in-the-blank, true or false, multiple-choice, short-answer, labeling, case study, mind mapping, matching, drawing, collage, and at-a-glance activities. Some of these activity types will be familiar to you or are self-explanatory; however, directions for the more complicated ones are given below.

Case Study

In the **Case Study** activity, you apply what you have learned to a hypothetical real-world situation. You may be asked to describe a solution or process that you would recommend for the case at hand. Case studies are answered in writing and typically require a paragraph-sized response.

Collage

In a **Collage**, you create a visual that responds to a given concept or prompt, either in the space provided or on a separate piece of paper or card. Find words, phrases, and pictures from magazines or the Internet and bring them together by printing and cutting them out and then taping, gluing, or stapling them to your canvas. Or, make a digital collage by copying and pasting together words and images into one image or document. Your instructor will provide guidance on how the class should complete their collages, including whether or not they will be displayed.

Labeling

The **Labeling** activity asks you to fill in the missing elements of a diagram or image from your textbook. Terms should be written at the end of the provided lines.

Rubrics

A **rubric** is a scoring document used to help you determine your level of development in a specific skill performance or behavior. A rubric is provided in the practical skills chapters of this workbook as a self-assessment tool to aid you in your behavior development. For every step in the procedure, choose *needs work or competent. Needs work* means you skipped the step or assistance is needed from your instructor and practice is needed to master the skill. *Competent* means the task is completed alone; performance includes rare errors. Space is provided for comments to assist you in improving your performance and achieving a higher rating.

Mind Mapping

Mind Mapping is a method you can use to create a visual representation of a concept or group of connected ideas. Basic guidelines for mind mapping a topic include the following:

*   Write the main topic or problem in the center of a piece of paper. Mind mapping activities in this workbook will do this first step for you.

*   Think about the topic and allow your ideas to flow.

- Write down key words or ideas that come to mind.
- Use lines to connect the key words to the main topic.
- Expand on the key words by creating new connections to additional thoughts or information.
- Use colors and/or symbols to highlight important information.

Refer to the completed Mind Map below a a helpful reference.

Best of luck to you from Milady!

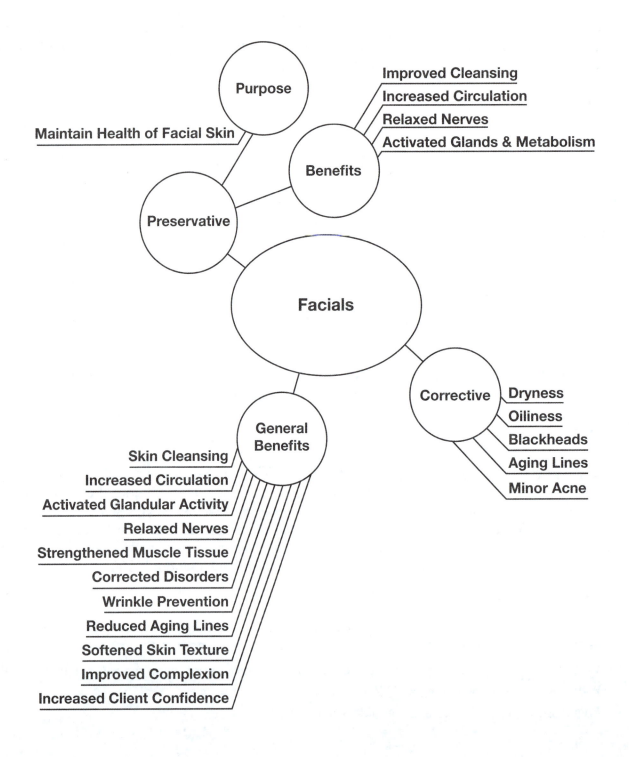

CHAPTER 1
CAREER OPPORTUNITIES AND HISTORY OF ESTHETICS

EXPLAIN HOW CAREER OPPORTUNITIES AND THE HISTORY OF THE PROFESSION ARE CRITICAL TO ESTHETICS

SHORT ANSWER

1. Why should estheticians study the history of esthetics?

_____

_____

_____

_____

_____

DESCRIBE THE CAREER OPTIONS AVAILABLE TO LICENSED ESTHETICIANS

SHORT ANSWER/MATCHING/MIND MAPPING

2. What is an esthetician, and what does an esthetician do?

_____

_____

_____

_____

_____

3. Match the career to its duties.

   a. salon or day spa esthetician

   b. clinical esthetician

   c. waxing specialist/brow specialist

   d. makeup artist

   e. manufacturer's representative

   f. salesperson or sales manager

   g. cosmetics buyer

   h. esthetics writer or beauty editor

   i. travel industry

   j. educator

   k. product development

   l. state licensing inspector or examiner

   m. state board member

   n. oncology-trained esthetician

   _____ performs advanced treatments, including laser and light therapies

   _____ capable and skillful in removing all face and body hair

   _____ writes intriguing articles/posts that are of interest and value to the esthetics community

   _____ has a full understanding of the industry and business and attends trade shows to keep up to date on new ingredients

   _____ performs facials and facial massage, waxing, and body treatments, applied both manually and with the aid of machines

   _____ has retail skills related to recommending makeup products and colors for home use; knowledgeable about the latest trends in color; efficient and creative

   _____ keeps up with the latest products and is able to recognize and anticipate trends in skin care

   _____ knows how and when to modify spa services for the safety of the client before, during, and after cancer treatments

   _____ calls on spas, salons, drugstores, department stores, and specialty businesses to help build clientele and increase product sales

   _____ develops lesson plans, curriculum, worksheets, tests, and any other supplements to assist in teaching others

   _____ performs esthetics services on cruise liners or in airports

   _____ assists in developing laws that will protect the public

   _____ keeps records of sales and stock on hand, demonstrates products, and sells to clients

   _____ conducts regular salon and spa inspections to ensure that managers and employees are following state rules and regulations and meeting ethical standards

MIND MAPPING

4. Mind mapping simply creates a free-flowing outline of material or information with the central or key point being located in the center. (Refer to How to Use this Workbook for more details on how to create a mind map.) Diagram the different career opportunities awaiting you upon your completion of your training. Identify the different disciplines and branches of each, including the different positions that may be obtained in each field. Use terms, pictures, and symbols as desired. Using color will increase the mind's retention and memory of the information. Keep your mind open and uncluttered and don't worry about where a line or word should go. The organization of the map will usually take care of itself.

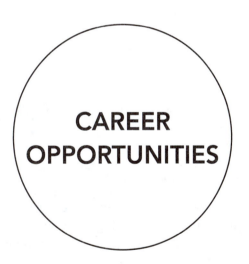

LIST TYPES OF EXISTING ESTHETICS PRACTICES TO CHART YOUR CAREER PATH

SHORT ANSWER

5. Choose one of the esthetics practices that you can see yourself working in. Describe its characteristics and why you like that practice type.

_____

_____

_____

_____

_____

6. Identify questions you may ask someone working in the esthetics practice that you are considering. It is great to have questions or topics prepared in case you have the opportunity to interview someone who is already established.

_____

_____

_____

_____

_____

OUTLINE SKIN CARE PRACTICES FROM EARLY CULTURES

COLLAGE/SHORT ANSWER

7. Using the material contained in the textbook and any other resources available to you, create a visual collage of the history of skin care from the beginning of its recorded history to the present. Identify interesting facts that are not already in the chapter. Be sure to indicate the year, decade, or century.

   Use drawings or pictures (cut and pasted) of products, people, tools, and implements that represent that era. Make a collage by taping, gluing, or stapling the words and images together. An alternative is to create the collage online, digitally combining the images gathered as one document.

8. Review your creation and choose a time period. Describe how that time period has influenced a current esthetics trend.

_____

_____

_____

_____

_____

SUMMARIZE THE CURRENT AND FUTURE STATES OF THE ESTHETICS INDUSTRY

SHORT ANSWER

9. Describe the current and future states of the esthetics industry. If you use resources other than your text, be sure to give credit to the source.

_____

_____

_____

_____

_____

WORD REVIEW

FILL IN THE BLANK

10. Provide the correct vocabulary term for each statement:

A dye obtained from the powdered leaves and shoots of the mignonette tree; used as a reddish hair dye and in tattooing is _____.

A(n) _____ is a specialist in the cleansing, beautification, and preservation of the health of the skin on the entire body, including the face and neck.

The integration of surgical procedures and esthetics treatments is _____.

_____ is the study and treatment of cancer and tumors.

A branch of anatomical science that deals with the overall health and well-being of the skin, the largest organ of the human body, is _____.

The Greek word meaning skilled in the use of cosmetics is _____.

DISCOVERIES AND ACCOMPLISHMENTS

In the space below, write notes about key concepts discussed in this chapter. Share your discoveries with some of the other students in your class and ask them if your notes are helpful. You may want to revise your discoveries based on good ideas shared by your peers.

Discoveries:

_____

_____

_____

_____

_____

_____

_____

_____

_____

_____

_____

_____

List at least three things you have accomplished that relate to your career goals.

Accomplishments:

_____

_____

_____

_____

_____

_____

_____

_____

_____

_____

_____

_____

EXAM REVIEW

MULTIPLE CHOICE

1. _____ is a career in which you can continuously learn new skills and make a difference in the health and well-being of the skin.

    a. Anesthesiology

    b. Esthetics

    c. Design

    d. Enthusiast

2. What is the largest organ of the human body?

    a. heart

    b. brain

    c. stomach

    d. skin

3. To make a diagnosis and prescribe medication, you need to be a(n) _____.

    a. dermatologist

    b. esthetician

    c. cosmetologist

    d. manicurist

4. What does a manufacturer's representative do?

    a. perform safety inspections

    b. train others on product knowledge and how to sell products

    c. perform esthetics treatments on clients

    d. sell products to customers

5. What was a bare (shaved or tweezed) eyebrow thought to signify during the Renaissance?

    a. greater social standing

    b. greater wealth

    c. greater intelligence

    d. greater fertility

6. A medical setting is where a _____ works.

    a. clinical esthetician

    b. salon or day spa esthetician

    c. waxing specialist

    d. makeup artist

7. Who purchases the products that are sold within a retail setting?

    a. manufacturer's representative

    b. salesperson

    c. cosmetic buyer

    d. beauty editor

8. A social media presence is typically a requirement for this position.

    a. manufacturer's representative

    b. salesperson

    c. cosmetic buyer

    d. beauty editor

9. What type of magnificent public buildings were the ancient Romans famous for constructing?

    a. smokehouses

    b. baths

    c. swimming pools

    d. massage parlors

10. Someone in which career needs to be prepared to conduct examinations, grant licenses, and inspect schools to see that certain physical standards, such as those for space and equipment, are maintained?

    a. educator

    b. travel industry professional

    c. state board member

    d. oncology-trained esthetician

11. _____ is a relatively new career path working with clients with cancer that has expanded quickly based on need.

    a. Educator

    b. Travel industry professional

    c. State board member

    d. Oncology-trained esthetician

12. During the Age of Extravagance, what did people color their lips and cheeks with?

   a. elderberry

   b. geranium petals

   c. camilla

   d. pomegranate

13. Which establishment is most appealing to those who appreciate working with a constantly changing clientele?

   a. franchised salon

   b. independently owned salon

   c. resort spa

   d. wellness center

14. What culture frequently bathed in olive oil?

   a. ancient Greeks

   b. ancient Romans

   c. ancient Egyptians

   d. ancient Asians

15. This culture used turmeric as a main ingredient in their facial masks to prevent wrinkles and skin discoloration.

   a. ancient Greeks

   b. ancient Romans

   c. ancient Egyptians

   d. ancient Asians

16. When was pale skin a sign of wealth and status?

   a. Middle Ages

   b. Renaissance era

   c. Roman age

   d. baby boomer era

17. In which time period did women pinch their cheeks and bite their lips to induce natural color rather than use cosmetics such as lipstick and rouge?

   a. Middle Ages

   b. Renaissance era

   c. Victorian age

   d. baby boomer era

18. Antioxidants and vitamins are part of which component of the esthetics industry?

    a. technology

    b. facilities/services

    c. consumers

    d. ingredients

19. These trends are all on the rise, except for _____.

    a. minimally invasive technology

    b. products containing gluten

    c. men's skin care

    d. retirement centers

20. A wellness center or spa _____.

    a. focuses on the health benefits or age-management aspect of skin care

    b. provides a total beauty experience, including hair services, makeup artistry, and nail and skin care

    c. is an amenity spa that provides guests with a variety of spa services that may include skin care, massage, and hair and nail services

    d. may offer a combination of other holistic health practices similar to those available at a skin care clinic or day spa

CHAPTER 2
ANATOMY AND PHYSIOLOGY

EXPLAIN WHY ESTHETICIANS NEED KNOWLEDGE OF ANATOMY AND PHYSIOLOGY

SHORT ANSWER

1. As an esthetics professional, an overview of human anatomy and physiology is part of your studies and allows you to be more effective in the services you provide. What do you think the importance of anatomy and physiology is to your career as an esthetician? Provide your answer on the lines below.

_____

_____

_____

_____

_____

_____

_____

_____

_____

_____

_____

_____

_____

_____

_____

_____

_____

_____

MATCHING

2. Match the following terms with their definitions: **anatomy, physiology, histology**

_____ the study of the structure and composition of tissue, also known as microscopic anatomy

_____ the study of the structures of the human body and substances these structures are made of; the science of the interconnected detail of organisms or of their parts

_____ the study of the functions and activities performed by the body structures, including physical and chemical processes

DESCRIBE THE BASIC STRUCTURE AND FUNCTION OF A CELL

SHORT ANSWER

3. Cells are the basic unit of all living things. What are they responsible for?

_____

_____

_____

_____

_____

Basic Structure of the Cell

LABELING

4. Label the cell diagram with the following terms: nucleus, mitochondria, and cell membrane.

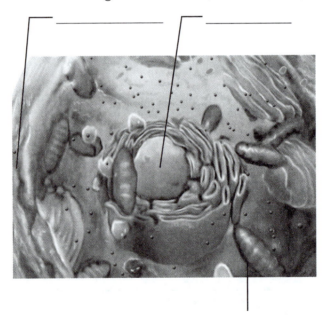

_____   _____

_____

SHORT ANSWER

5. Write a brief summary describing the function of each cell structure.

nucleus

_____

_____

_____

_____

_____

protoplasm

_____
_____
_____
_____
_____

mitochondria

_____
_____
_____
_____
_____

cell membrane

_____
_____
_____
_____
_____

Cell Reproduction and Division and Metabolism

FILL IN THE BLANK

6. Cell reproduction provides new cells for the _____ and _____ of worn or injured ones.

7. _____ is the normal process of cell reproduction in human tissues that occurs when the cell _____ into two identical cells called _____.

8. Favorable conditions for cell growth and reproduction include an adequate supply of _____, oxygen, and water; suitable _____; and the ability to eliminate _____.

9. _____, a chemical process that takes place in living organisms, converts nutrients to _____ so the cell can function and eliminates waste.

SHORT ANSWER

10. Explain why understanding the cell's metabolism is important as an esthetician.

_____

_____

_____

_____

_____

DESCRIBE THE FOUR TYPES OF TISSUE FOUND IN THE BODY

ESSAY

11. List and define the four types of tissues.

_____

_____

_____

_____

_____

_____

_____

_____

_____

DEFINE THE FUNCTIONS OF MAJOR ORGANS AND SYSTEMS OF THE BODY THAT INTERSECT WITH THE INTEGUMENTARY SYSTEM AND ESTHETICS

SHORT ANSWER

12. Tissues make up organs and organs make up systems. The body systems engage certain organs that perform a specific function. There are 11 major systems in the body. Identify the body system that matches its function.

_____ controls movement of blood throughout the body

_____ breaks down food into nutrients or waste for nutrition or excretion

_____ controls hormone levels that determine growth, development, sexual function, and health of entire body

_____ eliminates waste from the body, reducing buildup of toxins

_____ provides protective covering and regulates body temperature

_____ protects the body from disease by developing immunity and destroying pathogens and toxins

_____ covers, shapes, and holds the skeleton in place; contracts and moves various parts of the body

_____ coordinates with all other body systems, allowing them to work efficiently and react to the environment; carries messages

_____ produces offspring and allows for transfer of genetic material; differentiates between the sexes

_____ makes blood and oxygen available to body structures through breathing; eliminates carbon dioxide

_____ forms the physical foundation of the body; consists of bones that are connected by moveable and immovable joints

LIST THE FIVE ACCESSORY ORGANS TO THE SKIN

SHORT ANSWER

13. List the five accessory organs to the skin.

_____

_____

_____

_____

_____

IDENTIFY THE FIVE FUNCTIONS OF THE SKELETAL SYSTEM

SHORT ANSWER

14. Define the skeletal system and explain why it is important to understand as an esthetician.

_____

_____

_____

_____

_____

The Number of Bones and Composition

FILL IN THE BLANK

15. The adult skeleton has _____ bones that form a rigid framework.

16. _____ are connected to bones by tendons. Bones are connected to _____ by ligaments.

17. The connection between two or more bones of the skeleton is called a _____. There are two types: _____ and _____.

Functions

SHORT ANSWER

18. List the five primary functions of the skeletal system:

a) _____

b) _____

c) _____

d) _____

e) _____

Bones of the Skull, Face, Neck, Chest, Arms, and Hands

FILL IN THE BLANK

19. The skull is divided into two parts: the _____ and the _____.

20. The main bones of the neck include the _____, which supports the tongue and its muscles, and the _____, the seven bones of the top part of the vertebral column.

LABELING

21. Label the bones of the cranium.

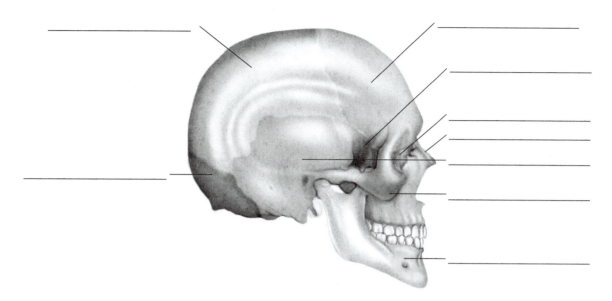

22. Label the bones of the face.

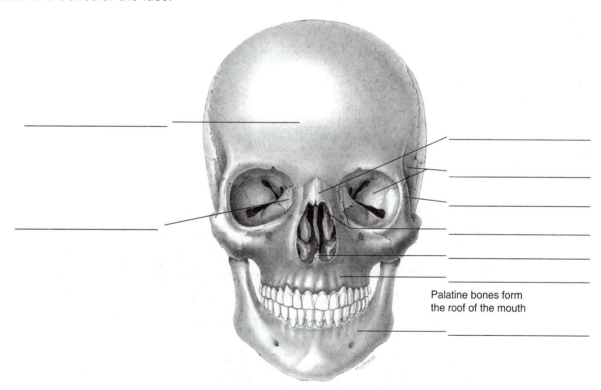

Palatine bones form
the roof of the mouth

23. Using the words from the following word bank, label the various parts of the diagram.

clavicle	sternum	ribs
scapula	thorax	

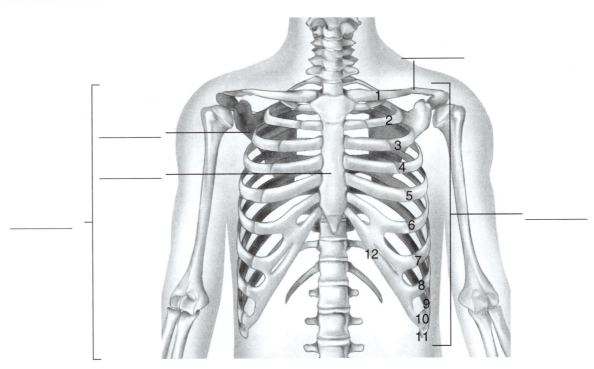

24. Using the words from the following word bank, label the various parts of the diagram.

humerus	phalanges	carpus	clavicle
radius	ulna	metacarpus	scapula

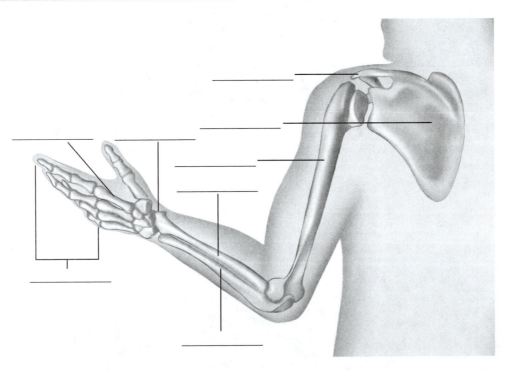

RECOGNIZE THE MUSCLES INVOLVED IN ESTHETIC MASSAGE

SHORT ANSWER

Answer the following questions in the spaces provided.

25. What are the main functions of the muscular system?

a) _____

b) _____

26. Why is having knowledge of the muscular system important as an esthetician?

_____

_____

_____

_____

_____

The Number of Muscles and Composition

FILL IN THE BLANK

27. The body has more than 630 muscles, which account for approximately ____ percent of its weight.

28. What are the three types of muscle tissue?

a) _____

b) _____

c) _____

29. List the three parts of a skeletal muscle and their location in relation to the skeleton.

a) _____

b) _____

c) _____

30. Pressure in massage is usually directed from the _____ to the _____.

31. List the treatments in which muscular tissue can be positively influenced.

a) _____

b) _____

c) _____

d) _____

e) _____

Muscles of the Scalp, Eyebrow, Nose, Mouth, Mastication, Ear, and Neck

FILL IN THE BLANK

32. Identify the group to which each muscle belongs.

   a) orbicularis oris: _____

   b) orbicularis oculi: _____

   c) frontalis: _____

   d) platysma: _____

   e) auricularis posterior: _____

   f) procerus: _____

   g) sternocleidomastoid (SCM): _____

   h) masseter: _____

   i) occipitalis: _____

   j) buccinator: _____

   k) nasalis: _____

   l) corrugator: _____

   m) temporalis: _____

LABELING

33. Label the muscles of the eyebrow.

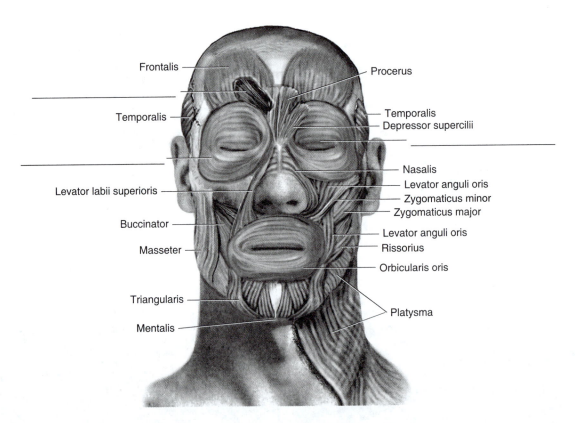

Muscles That Attach the Arms to the Body and Muscles of Shoulder and Arm

MATCHING

34. Match each of these muscles in the chest, shoulder or arm to its description.

a. deltoid	c. triceps	e. biceps
b. trapezius	d. pectoralis major	f. latissimus dorsi

_____ large, flat triangular muscle that covers the lower back

_____ muscle producing the contour of the front and inner side of the upper arm; lifts the forearm, flexes the elbow, and turns palm outward

_____ muscle of the chest that assists in the swinging movements of the arm

_____ large muscle that covers the entire back of the upper arm and extends the forearm

_____ muscle that covers the back of the neck, shoulders, and upper and middle region of the back; shrugs the shoulders and stabilizes the scapula

_____ large triangular muscle covering the shoulder joint; allows arm to extend outward and to the side of the body

LABELING

35. Label the muscles of the shoulders and upper arms.

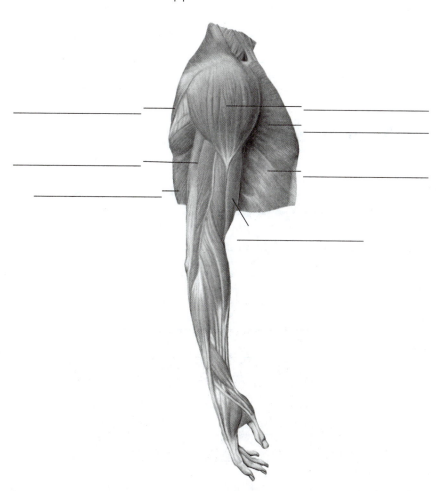

TRUE OR FALSE

36. For the following statements on muscle movements, circle T if true or F if false.

    T   F   Flexion is when your wrist, hand, and fingers straighten to form a line.

    T   F   Pronation is when muscles turn outward.

    T   F   When you draw your fingers together, you use adductor muscles.

    T   F   When bent over, you use your extensor muscles to stand up straight.

    T   F   Abduction separates the toes.

    T   F   You use your supinator muscles when turning your palm upward.

DESCRIBE THE THREE NERVE BRANCHES OF THE HEAD, NECK, AND FACE ESSENTIAL FOR PERFORMING FACIAL TREATMENTS

SHORT ANSWER

37. How will knowledge of the nervous system enhance your career as an esthetician?

_____

_____

_____

_____

_____

Divisions of the Nervous System

SHORT ANSWER

38. Describe the three main subdivisions of the nervous system.

    a)   the central nervous system: _____

    _____

    _____

    _____

    b)   the peripheral nervous system: _____

    _____

    _____

    _____

c) the autonomic nervous system: _____

_____

_____

_____

_____

The Brain and Spinal Cord

FILL IN THE BLANK

39. The _____ is the largest and most complex mass of nerve tissue in the body. It sends and receives messages through _____ pairs of cranial nerves that reach various parts of the head, face, and neck.

40. The _____ originates in the brain, extends down to the lower extremity of the trunk, and is protected by the spinal column.

41. The _____ connects the spinal cord to the brain and is involved in vital functions like breathing, heartbeat, and blood pressure.

Nerve Cell Structure and Function

SHORT ANSWER

42. List the two types of nerves and describe how they carry impulses.

a) _____

_____

b) _____

_____

43. Emily is cooking dinner and accidentally places her hand on a hot burner. She swiftly draws her hand back when she feels the heat. Explain the reflex process that occurred.

_____

_____

_____

_____

_____

Nerves of the Head, Face, and Neck

SHORT ANSWER

44. There are 12 pairs of cranial nerves arising at the base of the brain and the brain stem that activate the muscles and sensory structure of the head and neck. An esthetician is primarily concerned with three nerves. List the three nerves and describe what they control.

a) _____

_____

b) _____

_____

c) _____

_____

LABELING

45. Label where the fifth, seventh, and eleventh nerves are and their branches for the missing labels.

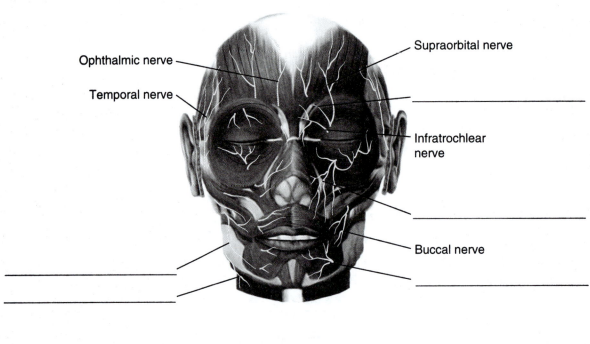

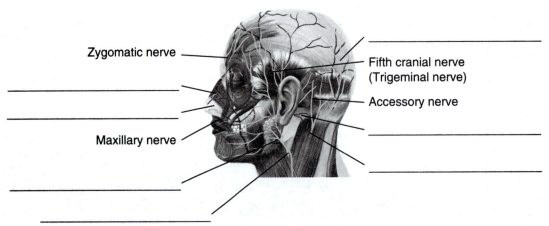

Nerves of the Arm and Hand

MATCHING

46. Match each of these sensory-motor nerves of the arm and hand to its description.

a. digital nerve	c. median nerve
b. radial nerve	d. ulnar nerve

_____ affects the little-finger side of the arm and palm of the hand

_____ smaller nerve than others that supplies the arm and hand

_____ supplies the thumb side of the arm and back of the hand

_____ supplies the fingers

SHORT ANSWER

47. Explain where the vagus nerve is located and why it is important to understand as an esthetician, especially during massage treatments.

_____

_____

_____

_____

_____

OUTLINE HOW THE CIRCULATORY SYSTEM INFLUENCES THE HEALTH OF THE SKIN

SHORT ANSWER

48. What is the primary function of the circulatory system? Explain why it is important to esthetics.

_____

_____

_____

_____

The Heart and Blood Vessels

SHORT ANSWER

49. Name the two systems that ensure continuous circulation and explain where they carry blood.

a) _____

_____

b) _____

_____

50. What is the function of the heart? _____ .

    Define the following terms.

    a) arteries: _____

    _____

    b) capillaries: _____

    _____

    c) veins: _____

    _____

    d) arterioles: _____

    _____

    e) venules: _____

    _____

The Blood

FILL IN THE BLANK

51. Blood is the _____ fluid circulating through the circulatory system and is considered _____ tissue.

52. There are _____ pints of blood in the human body.

53. The normal temperature of blood is _____ degrees Fahrenheit.

54. Name five critical functions of blood.

    a) _____

    b) _____

    _____

    c) _____

    d) _____

    _____

    e) _____

MATCHING

55. Match each component of blood to its description.

    | a. red blood cells | c. platelets |
    | b. white blood cells | d. plasma |

    _____ contribute to the blood-clotting process

    _____ carry oxygen to the body cells

    _____ carries vital components to the cells and takes waste away

    _____ destroy disease-causing microorganisms

Arteries and Veins of the Head, Face, and Neck

TRUE OR FALSE

56. For the following statements, circle T if true or F if false.

T   F   Common carotid arteries are located on either side of the neck.

T   F   The jugular veins are the main source of blood supply to the head, face, and neck.

T   F   Internal and external jugular veins run parallel to the carotid arteries.

T   F   Knowing facial vessel locations is important to avoid bruising during treatments.

EXPLAIN THE INTERDEPENDENCE OF THE LYMPHATIC, CIRCULATORY, AND IMMUNE SYSTEMS

SHORT ANSWER

57. The lymphatic system is closely connected to the circulatory system for the transportation of fluids. Describe how the lymphatic system is different.

_____

_____

_____

_____

_____

58. Explain the four primary functions of the lymphatic system.

a) _____

b) _____

c) _____

d) _____

59. Understanding the lymphatic and immune systems is very important when treating the skin. Explain why.

_____

_____

_____

_____

_____

IDENTIFY THE GLANDS THAT MAKE UP THE ENDOCRINE SYSTEM

SHORT ANSWER

60. Explain in your own words the endocrine system, endocrine glands, and all the glands within the system.

endocrine system: _____

_____

endocrine glands: _____

_____

The following glands are within the endocrine system.

a) _____

_____

b) _____

_____

c) _____

_____

d) _____

_____

e) _____

_____

f) _____

_____

g) _____

_____

LIST HOW HORMONAL CHANGES IN THE REPRODUCTIVE SYSTEM CAN AFFECT THE SKIN

SHORT ANSWER

61. What parts of the body are included in the reproductive system?

_____

_____

_____

_____

_____

62. The reproductive system produces hormones—estrogen in females and testosterone in males. These hormones, or lack thereof, affect and change the skin in several ways as we age. List the ways hormones could affect the body.

_____

_____

_____

_____

_____

_____

DESCRIBE WHAT OCCURS DURING INHALATION AND EXHALATION

FILL IN THE BLANK

63. The _____ system enables breathing, is located within the chest cavity, and is protected on both sides by the ribs.

64. The _____ are spongy tissues composed of microscopic cells in which inhaled air is exchanged for _____ in one breath.

65. The muscular wall that separates the thorax from the abdominal region and helps control breathing is called the _____.

SHORT ANSWER

66. Describe the breathing cycle.

_____

_____

_____

_____

_____

EXPLAIN THE FIVE STEPS IN DIGESTION

MATCHING

67. Match the term with the correct definition.

a. peristalsis	d. absorption	f. digestive enzymes
b. ingestion	e. defecation	g. digestive system
c. digestion		

_____ elimination of feces from the body

_____ moving food along the digestive tract

_____ the transport of fully digested food into the circulatory system to feed the tissues and cells

_____ breakdown of food by mechanical and chemical means

_____ responsible for breaking down foods into nutrients and wastes; consists of the mouth, stomach, intestines, salivary and gastric glands, and other organs

_____ eating or taking food into the body

_____ chemicals that change certain kinds of food into a form that can be used by the body

LIST THE FIVE ORGANS THAT COMPRISE THE EXCRETORY SYSTEM

FILL IN THE BLANK

The body has various organs that remove waste products before they become toxic.

68. The kidneys excrete _____.

69. The liver discharges _____.

70. The skin eliminates salts and minerals through _____.

71. The large intestine eliminates _____.

72. The lungs exhale _____.

WORD REVIEW

FILL IN THE BLANK

73. Provide the correct vocabulary term for each:

_____ the transport of fully digested food into the circulatory system to feed the tissues and cells

_____ middle part of a muscle

_____ muscles that draw a body part, such as a finger, arm, or toe, away from the midline of the body or of an extremity; in the hand, these separate the fingers

_____ also known as the collarbone; bone joining the sternum and scapula

_____ automatic nerve reaction to a stimulus; involves the movement of an impulse from a sensory receptor along the afferent nerve to the spinal cord, and a responsive impulse back along an efferent neuron to a muscle, causing a reaction

_____ eating or taking food into the body

_____ main organs of the respiratory system in which inhaled air is exchanged for carbon dioxide during one respiratory cycle

_____ thin-walled blood vessels that connect the smaller arteries to the veins

_____ a specialized connective tissue considered fat, which gives smoothness and contour to the body and cushions and insulates the body

_____ condition of the skin that is triggered by hormones; causes darker pigmentation in areas such as the upper lip and around the eyes and cheeks

_____ hindmost bone of the skull; forms the back of the skull above the nape

_____ u-shaped bone at the base of the tongue that supports the tongue and its muscle

_____ smaller bone in the forearm on the same side as the thumb

_____ colorless watery fluid derived from blood plasma that protects the body from disease by developing a resistance to the microorganism

_____ external protective coating that covers the body; the body's largest organ; acts as a barrier to protect body systems from the outside elements

_____ muscle of the forearm that rotates the radius outward and the palm upward

_____ chest; elastic, bony cage that serves as a protective framework for the heart, lungs, and other internal organs

_____ muscle producing the contour of the front and inner side of the upper arm

_____ collection of similar cells that perform a particular function

_____ inner and larger bone of the forearm; attached to the wrist on the side of the little finger

_____ thick-walled muscular, flexible tubes that carry oxygenated blood from the heart to the capillaries throughout the body

_____ carry impulses or messages from the sense organs to the brain where sensations are experienced

_____ the normal process of cell reproduction of human tissues; cells dividing into two new identical daughter cells

DISCOVERIES AND ACCOMPLISHMENTS

In the space below, write notes about key concepts discussed in this chapter. Share your discoveries with some of the other students in your class and ask them if your notes are helpful. You may want to revise your discoveries based on good ideas shared by your peers.

Discoveries:

_____

_____

_____

_____

_____

_____

_____

_____

_____

_____

_____

_____

List at least three things you have accomplished that relate to your career goals.

Accomplishments:

_____

_____

_____

_____

_____

_____

_____

_____

_____

_____

_____

EXAM REVIEW

MULTIPLE CHOICE

1. How much blood does the human body contain?

    a. one to three pints

    b. eight to 10 pints

    c. 12 to 14 pints

    d. 17 to 20 pints

2. What is a nutritive fluid flowing through the circulatory system?

    a. lymph

    b. blood

    c. pus

    d. water

3. What are platelets?

    a. blood components that contribute to the blood clotting process

    b. a type of white blood cell

    c. a type of red blood cell

    d. dangerous bacteria found in the bloodstream

4. What is the study of tiny structures found in living tissues?

    a. anatomy

    b. physiology

    c. histology

    d. osteology

5. What is one reason estheticians should study body systems, organs, and tissues?

    a. to obtain the medical license needed to become an esthetician

    b. to perform emergency surgery in the salon

    c. to prescribe medications for clients with skin disorders

    d. to understand the effect that services have on the body

6. What is protoplasm?

    a. foundation of all chemical beauty products

    b. substance of which the cells of all living things are composed

    c. toxic substance found in the bodies of people with diseases

    d. yellowish fluid that oozes from open sores

7. What is the process of cell reproduction called?

    a. anagen

    b. catagen

    c. mitosis

    d. metastasization

8. What is the sternum?

    a. flat bone that forms the ventral support of the ribs

    b. uppermost bone of the skull

    c. longest bone in the foot

    d. collarbone

9. What is the fluid part of the blood that carries food and secretions to the cells and carbon dioxide from the cells?

    a. pus

    b. lymph

    c. plasma

    d. sebum

10. What is true of the origin part of a muscle?

    a. It is not attached to the skeleton.

    b. It disappears after puberty.

    c. It moves frequently.

    d. It is attached to the skeleton.

11. What are the structures composed of specialized tissues and performing specific functions?

    a. cells

    b. organs

    c. body systems

    d. bodies

12. Why does the parathyroid gland regulate blood calcium and phosphorous levels?

    a. so the endocrine and muscular systems can function properly

    b. so the nervous and muscular systems can function properly

    c. so the nervous and circulatory systems can function properly

    d. so the endocrine and circulatory systems can function properly

13. What is true of the pituitary gland?

     a. It is the most complex organ of the endocrine system.

     b. It is the most complex organ of the integumentary system.

     c. It has no effect on the physiological processes of the body.

     d. It affects very few of the body's physiological processes.

14. What organ in the endocrine system secretes enzyme-producing cells that are responsible for digesting carbohydrates, proteins, and fats?

     a. pancreas

     b. kidney

     c. liver

     d. stomach

15. What are the secretions that the endocrine glands release directly into the bloodstream and that influence the welfare of the entire body?

     a. red blood cells

     b. white blood cells

     c. endorphins

     d. hormones

16. What is the primary function of the respiratory system?

     a. digestion

     b. blood circulation

     c. reproduction

     d. breathing

17. What is the primary function of the lymphatic/immune system?

     a. protecting the body from disease

     b. providing the body's outer shell

     c. facilitating reproduction

     d. facilitating respiration

18. What is the primary function of the skeletal system?

     a. providing the exterior protective covering of the body

     b. circulating blood to the bones and to muscles attached to bones

     c. circulating oxygen to the bones and to muscles attached to bones

     d. providing the physical foundation of the body

19. What is the primary function of the circulatory system?
    a. promoting sebum production
    b. providing a path for waste products to move out of the body
    c. providing carbon dioxide to all cells of the body
    d. moving blood through the body

20. What is covered, shaped, and supported by the muscular system?
    a. integumentary system
    b. skeletal tissue
    c. vital organs
    d. secondary organs

21. What body system is responsible for changing food into nutrients and waste?
    a. endocrine
    b. integumentary
    c. excretory
    d. digestive

22. What is the primary function of the excretory system?
    a. purifying the body by elimination of waste matter
    b. converting food into nutrients and waste
    c. circulating blood and lymph throughout the body
    d. circulating nitrogen and oxygen throughout the body

23. What is the primary function of the reproductive system?
    a. discharging waste from the body
    b. perpetuating the human race
    c. maintaining erogenous zones
    d. feeding nutrients into the body

24. What is the body system that controls and coordinates all other body systems?
    a. endocrine
    b. reproductive
    c. integumentary
    d. nervous

25. What is a connection between two or more bones of the skeleton?
    a. joint
    b. ligament
    c. origin
    d. insertion

26. What body system serves as a protective covering for the body?

    a. endocrine

    b. skeletal

    c. nervous

    d. integumentary

27. Connective, epithelial, muscle, and nerve are types of what found in the body?

    a. lymph

    b. sebum

    c. body system

    d. tissue

28. What are valves?

    a. structures that close a passage or permit flow in one direction only

    b. exterior openings on the body such as aural canals, nostrils, and pores

    c. junctures in the digestive system where food is halted and processed

    d. junctures in the excretory system where waste is halted and processed

29. What bone forms the back of the skull above the nape?

    a. temporal

    b. occipital

    c. sphenoid

    d. ethmoid

30. How many identical daughter cells are formed when a cell divides during mitosis?

    a. two

    b. four

    c. six

    d. eight

31. What body system affects the growth, development, sexual activities, and health of the body?

    a. circulatory

    b. integumentary

    c. nervous

    d. endocrine

32. Where in the body does the spinal cord originate?
    a. top of the skull
    b. base of the neck
    c. brain
    d. heart

33. What are glands?
    a. sexual organs required for reproduction
    b. specialized organs that remove and convert elements from the blood
    c. chambers of the heart required for circulation
    d. groups of cells in the skin responsible for perspiration

34. What is the importance of lymph?
    a. to secrete enzymes necessary for digestion
    b. to synthesize proteins
    c. to fight infections
    d. to disperse white blood cells and cell nutrients

35. What binds the tissues of the body together?
    a. anatomical binders
    b. physiological binders
    c. adhesive tissue
    d. connective tissue

36. What carries messages to and from the brain and controls and coordinates all body functions?
    a. epithelial tissue
    b. cardiac tissue
    c. nerve tissue
    d. supervisory tissue

37. What organ circulates the blood?
    a. brain
    b. heart
    c. liver
    d. kidney

38. What do the kidneys do?
    a. pump nitrogen into the blood
    b. pump oxygen into the blood
    c. convert food to nutrients
    d. excrete water and waste products

39. Which of the following best completes the statement below? As one of the major body organs the brain has the function of _____.

    a. controlling the body's vision

    b. controlling the body

    c. supplying oxygen to the blood

    d. digesting food

40. What is defecation?

    a. circulating water through the body

    b. breaking food down into nutrients

    c. absorbing nutrients into the body

    d. eliminating waste from the body

41. Which body system controls and coordinates all bodily functions?

    a. skeletal

    b. nervous

    c. muscular

    d. circulatory

42. Which body system regulates temperature and produces vitamin D?

    a. integumentary

    b. skeletal

    c. muscular

    d. circulatory

43. Which body system protects the body from disease by developing resistances and destroying disease-causing toxins?

    a. endocrine

    b. circulatory

    c. immune/lymphatic

    d. reproductive

44. Which body system eliminates carbon dioxide as a waste product?

    a. endocrine

    b. circulatory

    c. respiratory

    d. reproductive

45. The kidneys and bladder are part of this system.

    a. excretory

    b. digestive

    c. respiratory

    d. immune/lymphatic

46. Which type of muscle will estheticians work with?

    a. smooth

    b. cardiac

    c. skeletal

    d. involuntary

47. Which part of the muscle flexes but remains stationary?

    a. belly

    b. origin

    c. insertion

    d. smooth

48. Which muscle draws the scalp backward?

    a. frontalis

    b. corrugator

    c. occipitalis

    d. epicranial aponeurosis

49. Which muscle causes wrinkles in the forehead?

    a. frontalis

    b. orbicularis oculi

    c. occipitalis

    d. mentalis

50. This muscle closes the eyes.

    a. corrugator

    b. orbicularis oculi

    c. procerus

    d. epicranial aponeurosis

51. Which thin, flat muscle between the upper and lower jaws compresses the cheeks and expels air between the lips?

    a. mentalis

    b. triangularis

    c. buccinator

    d. risorius

52. This muscle pulls down the corners of the mouth.

    a. mentalis

    b. triangularis

    c. buccinator

    d. risorius

53. If you want to pucker up, you need to use the _____ muscle.

    a. obicularis oris

    b. levator anguli oris

    c. levator labii superioris

    d. zygomaticus

54. You use this muscle to smile, but not grin.

    a. obicularis oris

    b. levator anguli oris

    c. levator labii superioris

    d. nasalis

55. This muscle is used to grin.

    a. mentalis

    b. triangularis

    c. buccinator

    d. risorius

56. Which of these muscles are used in chewing?

    a. levator anguli oris and levator labii superioris

    b. zygomaticus and risorius

    c. masseter and temporalis

    d. triangularis and buccinator

57. What are the three muscles of the ear called?

    a. quadratus labii muscles

    b. depressor anguli muscles

    c. mastication muscles

    d. auricularis muscles

58. When you turn your head, you are using the _____ muscle.

    a. sternocleidomastoid

    b. platysma

    c. auricularis superior

    d. zygomaticus

59. Which large, flat, triangular muscle covers the lower back?

     a. sternocleidomastoid

     b. platysma

     c. latissimus dorsi

     d. pectoralis

60. When you show someone your muscles on your arm, you are most likely showing them your _____.

     a. biceps

     b. triceps

     c. deltoid

     d. trapezius

61. Which movement separates the fingers?

     a. abduction

     b. adduction

     c. flexion

     d. extension

62. When you bend forward, which muscle movement are you using?

     a. abduction

     b. adduction

     c. flexion

     d. extension

63. This movement is used to rotate the muscles.

     a. abduction

     b. extension

     c. flexion

     d. supination

64. How does massage help the muscles of the hand?

     a. maintains good body mechanics

     b. maintains pliability

     c. activates inward muscles

     d. rotates radials

65. Why is it important as an esthetician to know about the muscles of the forearm?

     a. to maintain good body mechanics

     b. to maintain pliability

     c. to activate inward muscles

     d. to rotate radials

CHAPTER 3
PHYSIOLOGY AND HISTOLOGY OF THE SKIN

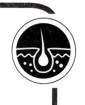

DESCRIBE WHY LEARNING THE PHYSIOLOGY AND HISTOLOGY OF THE SKIN MAKES YOU A BETTER ESTHETICIAN

SHORT ANSWER

1. Why do you think estheticians should have a thorough understanding of the physiology and histology of the skin?

_____

_____

_____

_____

_____

_____

_____

_____

_____

_____

DESCRIBE THE ATTRIBUTES OF HEALTHY SKIN

FILL IN THE BLANK

2. Four descriptors of healthy skin are:

- _____
- _____
- _____
- _____

DISTINGUISH THE SIX PRIMARY FUNCTIONS OF THE SKIN

TRUE OR FALSE

3. For the following statements about the skin, circle T if true or F if false:

    T   F   It acts as an insulator to protect the body from extreme heat and cold.

    T   F   It aids in bone health by producing vitamin C.

    T   F   It is a sensory storehouse.

    T   F   It allows chemicals and bacteria into our system.

Sensation

SHORT ANSWER

4. What kind of sensations can nerve sensors detect?

    _____

    _____

    _____

    _____

    _____

Protection

MATCHING

5. Match the term to the correct statement.

a. hydrolipidic film	e. acid mantle
b. barrier function	f. fibroblasts
c. transepidermal water loss	g. epidermal growth factor
d. intercellular matrix	

    _____ skin's mechanism that protects from irritation and dehydration

    _____ water loss caused by evaporation on the skin's surface

    _____ average pH of 5.5; part of the skin's natural barrier function

    _____ hormone that stimulates skin cells to reproduce and heal

    _____ protects the skin from drying out and exposure to external factors

    _____ lipid substances that protect cells from water loss and irritation

    _____ cell stimulators that are triggered by proteins and peptides

Heat Regulation

FILL IN THE BLANK

6. The body's average internal thermostat is set at _____ degrees Fahrenheit.

7. The body maintains thermoregulation through _____, _____, _____, and _____.

8. Sometimes the terms _____ and _____ are used interchangeably.

9. _____ are tubelike depressions with oil glands attached to them.

10. _____ are tubelike openings for sweat glands on the epidermis.

11. When we are cold, the _____ attached to the hair follicles contract and cause "goosebumps."

Excretion

SHORT ANSWER

12. Describe what happens when you sweat.

_____

_____

_____

_____

_____

Secretion

FILL IN THE BLANK

13. _____ are appendages attached to follicles that produce _____, an oily substance that protects the surface of the skin.

14. Acneic breakouts can be caused by an increased flow of sebum because of stimulation of the oil glands due to emotional stress or _____.

Absorption

SHORT ANSWER

15. Describe how different sized molecules penetrate the skin.

_____

_____

_____

_____

_____

EXPLAIN THE FUNCTION OF EACH LAYER OF THE SKIN, FROM THE DEEPEST TO THE SURFACE

MATCHING

16. Match the term to the correct statements.

a. adipose tissue

b. dermis

c. reticular layer

d. hair papillae

e. keratin

f. epidermis

g. stratum corneum

h. melanin

i. collagen

j. elastin

k. lymph vessels

l. dermal/epidermal junction

m. stratum germinativum

n. stratum spinosum

o. stratum granulosum

p. stratum lucidum

q. melanocytes

r. glycosaminoglycans

_____ also called corium or true skin; consists of two layers and supplies skin with oxygen and nutrients

_____ fibrous protein that provides resiliency and protection to the skin

_____ thin, protective covering with many nerve endings; consists of five layers called strata

_____ large protein molecules and water-binding substances found between the fibers of the dermis

_____ where cells continue to divide and enzymes are creating lipids and proteins

_____ skin pigment

_____ horny layer of the epidermis

_____ fibrous protein that gives skin its strength and is necessary for wound healing

_____ cells that produce pigment granules in the basal layer

_____ where production of keratin and intercellular lipids take place

_____ remove waste products, bacteria, and excess fluid

_____ fibrous protein that forms elastic tissue and gives skin its elasticity

_____ thin, clear layer of dead skin cells

_____ consists of layers of a connective collagen tissue with many small pockets and holes

_____ subcutaneous layer composed of fat

_____ where stem cells undergo continuous mitosis to replenish skin cells that are shed from the surface

_____ denser and deeper layer of the dermis; comprised mainly of collagen and elastin

_____ small, cone-shaped structures at the bottom of hair follicles

IDENTIFY A HAIR FOLLICLE AS AN APPENDAGE OF THE SKIN

SHORT ANSWER

17. Explain how hair is an appendage of the skin and the importance of understanding this as an esthetician.

_____

_____

_____

_____

_____

18. How do hormones and genetics influence hair growth?

_____

_____

_____

_____

IDENTIFY NAILS AS AN APPENDAGE OF THE SKIN

TRUE OR FALSE

19. For the following statements about the nail, circle T if true or F if false:

T   F   Some symptoms of diseases and disorders that influence the skin are evident on the nails.

T   F   The nail is composed of soft keratin.

T   F   In some states, performing nail services is part of the scope of practice of an esthetician.

T   F   The nail plate contains nerves and blood vessels.

T   F   The technical term for the nail is nail plate.

T   F   Toenails grow faster than fingernails.

LABEL

20. Label the nail structure.

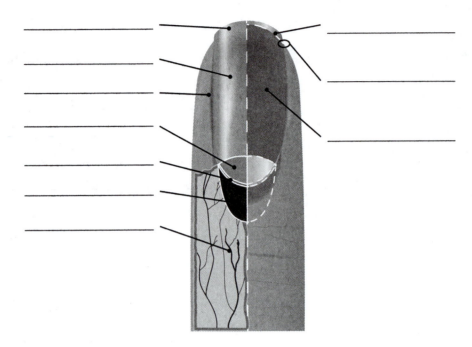

DESCRIBE THE FUNCTIONS OF THE TWO TYPES OF NERVES

SHORT ANSWER

21. List and describe the two types of nerves.

- _____
  _____
  _____
- _____
  _____
  _____

EXPLAIN WHAT IS PRODUCED BY THE TWO TYPES OF GLANDS OF THE SKIN

SHORT ANSWER

22. Name the two types of glands of the skin and what substance they produce.

- _____
- _____

23. What happens if the sebaceous gland ducts get clogged?

_____

_____

_____

24. While the oil produced by the sebaceous glands protects the surface of the skin, how do the sudoriferous glands help the body?

_____

_____

_____

25. Name the two kinds of sweat glands and explain how they are different.

- _____

  _____

  _____

  _____

- _____

  _____

  _____

  _____

DISTINGUISH THE FACTORS INFLUENCING SKIN HEALTH

SHORT ANSWER

26. What influences skin health and aging of the skin?

_____

_____

_____

_____

_____

MATCHING

27. Match the term to the correct statement.

a. Langerhans cells

b. free radicals

c. leukocytes

d. T cells

e. lipids

f. blood

g. cells

h. lymph

i. ceramides

j. UVA radiation

k. UVB radiation

l. UVC radiation

m. high-energy visible light

n. antioxidants

_____ attack virus-infected cells, foreign cells, and cancer cells

_____ a group of waxy lipid molecules that are important to barrier function

_____ penetrates deeper into the skin and causes genetic damage and cell death

_____ clear fluid of the body that bathes skin cells and removes toxins and cellular waste

_____ white blood cells that have enzymes to digest and kill bacteria and parasites

_____ reacts with the ozone high in our atmosphere

_____ components that have an extra electron and neutralize the chain reaction caused by free radicals

_____ are reduced if the skin is dry, damaged, or mature

_____ the body replaces billions of these daily

_____ is said to penetrate the skin more deeply than UV rays and damage collagen, hyaluronic acid, and elastin

_____ work to absorb, process, and carry antigens to the nearest lymph node for future immune system action

_____ supplies nutrients and oxygen to the skin

_____ causes burning of the skin as well as tanning, aging, and cancer

_____ unstable molecules that steal electrons from other molecules to regain balance

Skin Health and the Environment

SHORT ANSWER

28. List three environmental factors that can affect the skin.

- _____

- _____

- _____

29. What can you do to remove the buildup of pollutants on the skin and protect against them?

_____

_____

_____

_____

_____

_____

_____

_____

Skin Health and Lifestyle Choices

SHORT ANSWER

30. Describe how smoking and drinking alcoholic beverages influence the aging process.

_____

_____

_____

_____

_____

_____

_____

_____

Glycation

SHORT ANSWER

31. What is glycation and what causes this process?

_____

_____

_____

_____

_____

Aging Skin and Hormones

SHORT ANSWER

32. How does estrogen affect the skin?

_____

_____

_____

_____

_____

Microcirculation

FILL IN THE BLANK

33. Microcirculation is the circulation of blood from the heart to _____, to _____, to _____, and then back to the heart.

34. One cause of microcirculation problems in mature skin is _____.

35. _____ skin, or telangiectasia, is the dilation of the capillary walls and is one problem of microcirculation.

36. List three other causes of microcirculation.

- _____

- _____

- _____

Hormone Replacement Therapy

TRUE OR FALSE

37. For the following statements about the Hormone Replacement Therapy, circle T if true or F if false:

   T F   An esthetician should recommend HRT regimens.

   T F   HRT is often suggested to balance testosterone for women experiencing menopause.

   T F   Estrogens from plants are weaker than animal estrogens.

   T F   Estrogens from animals are called phytoestrogens.

   T F   Some HRT may be linked to breast cancer.

WORD REVIEW

WORD SEARCH

38. Answer the following questions and then find the word within the word search.

What is the technical name for a nail? _____

Hair and nails are made of the hard type of what? _____

Motor nerves, such as ones that stimulate the arrector pili muscles, are also known as which type of nerve? _____

Sensory nerves, such as ones that feel cold and heat, are also known as which type of nerve? _____

Which type of sudoriferous gland is attached to hair follicles and releases secretions through the oil glands? _____

Which type of sudoriferous gland is found all over the body, primarily the forehead, palms of the hands, and soles of the feet? _____

What is the protein substance of complex fibers that give skin its strength? _____

What is the process by which keratinocytes are continually shed from the skin? _____

What are the protein bonds, developed in the stratum spinosum, that create junctions between cells called? _____

What is another name for couperose skin? _____

What is the deepest layer of the skin called? _____

What is the name of the chronic vascular disorder where telangiectasia is visible? _____

What is the complex protein which determines skin, eye, and hair color called? _____

```
O   A   S   R   A   P   O   C   R   I   N   E   N   A
N   F   U   C   O   L   L   A   G   E   N   A   I   D
Y   F   B   O   M   E   L   A   N   I   N   S   E   Q
X   E   C   E   M   S   S   T   G   I   K   S   T   D
R   R   U   C   O   U   D   G   B   J   Q   M   E   P
O   E   T   C   T   G   G   A   N   U   G   S   I   E
S   N   A   R   H   A   W   T   A   Z   M   Q   F   M
A   T   N   I   I   N   R   M   P   O   A   F   B   C
C   Q   E   N   S   Q   A   L   S   J   E   N   Q   R
E   O   O   E   H   T   J   O   F   R   Y   K   R   C
A   H   U   A   I   H   M   Y   E   O   I   M   N   V
Z   I   S   O   C   E   R   N   Q   E   T   H   I   T
X   B   N   Q   S   W   T   K   E   R   A   T   I   N
T   E   L   A   N   G   I   E   C   T   A   S   I   A
```

DISCOVERIES AND ACCOMPLISHMENTS

In the space below, write notes about key concepts discussed in this chapter. Share your discoveries with some of the other students in your class and ask them if your notes are helpful. You may want to revise your discoveries based on good ideas shared by your peers.

Discoveries:

_____

_____

_____

_____

_____

_____

_____

_____

_____

_____

_____

_____

List at least three things you have accomplished since your last entry that relate to your career goals.

Accomplishments:

_____

_____

_____

_____

_____

_____

_____

_____

_____

_____

_____

_____

EXAM REVIEW

MULTIPLE CHOICE

1. Why is UVB radiation also known as "burning rays"?
    a. UVB wavelengths cause cancer as well as burning of the skin.
    b. UVB radiation burns paper upon direct exposure.
    c. UVB radiation burns wood upon direct exposure.
    d. UVB causes genetic damage and cell death.

2. What is not an element of the skin's acid mantle?
    a. blood
    b. sebum
    c. lipids
    d. sweat

3. What causes injured skin to restore itself to its normal thickness?
    a. hyperproduction of cells
    b. daily exposure to the sun
    c. gentle massage
    d. Botox injections

4. Histology is also known as _____.
    a. the study of body structures
    b. microscopic anatomy
    c. physical processes
    d. facial technology

5. Which of the following is not a characteristic of healthy skin?
    a. moist
    b. smooth
    c. slightly rough
    d. somewhat acidic

6. What are most abundant in the fingertips, as opposed to other parts of the body?
    a. red blood cells
    b. white blood cells
    c. lymph nodes
    d. sensory nerve fibers

7. What is the average internal temperature of the body in degrees Fahrenheit?

    a. 37

    b. 96.8

    c. 98.6

    d. 99.5

8. Why does the body perspire?

    a. to protect us from overheating

    b. to protect us from freezing

    c. to protect us from dehydration

    d. to protect us from overhydration

9. What are follicles?

    a. sweat gland openings

    b. tubelike openings in the epidermis

    c. tubelike openings in the muscles

    d. ingrown hair shafts

10. What is glycation?

    a. fibrous, connective tissue made from protein

    b. a white blood cell that has enzymes to digest and kill bacteria

    c. the binding of a protein molecule to a glucose molecule

    d. a chronic condition that appears primarily in the cheeks

11. What are hair papillae?

    a. ingrown hairs

    b. cone-shaped elevations at the base of the follicle

    c. shaved hairs

    d. membranes of ridges and grooves that attach to the epidermis

12. Where in the body is hyaluronic acid found?

    a. hair

    b. skin

    c. kidney

    d. liver

13.   What is hydrolipidic film?

    a.   salt–water balance that damages the skin's surface

    b.   oil–water balance that damages the skin's surface

    c.   salt–water balance that protects the skin's surface

    d.   oil–water balance that protects the skin's surface

14.   What is the acid mantle?

    a.   deposit left on the skin after the use of an acidic product

    b.   protective layer of lipids and secretions on the skin's surface

    c.   reservoir of digestive juices located in the stomach

    d.   deposit left on the skin after the use of an alkaline product

15.   Where in the body are the coiled structures known as apocrine glands found?

    a.   mouth and nostrils

    b.   underarm and genital areas

    c.   eyes and ears

    d.   lower back and inner knees

16.   What is the result of the contraction of the arrector pili muscle?

    a.   penile erection

    b.   excessive sweating

    c.   gaseous discharge

    d.   goosebumps

17.   What are ceramides?

    a.   glycolipid materials

    b.   hydrolipid materials

    c.   neurolipid materials

    d.   psycholipid materials

18.   What is collagen?

    a.   hardened keratinocyte

    b.   fibrous tissue made from protein

    c.   hydrating fluid found in the skin

    d.   pigment-carrying granule

19. What are corneocytes?
    a. open comedones
    b. hardened keratinocytes
    c. closed comedones
    d. softened keratinocytes

20. What are membranes of ridges and grooves that attach to the epidermis?
    a. follicular papillae
    b. dermal papillae
    c. epidermal papillae
    d. hair papillae

21. How fast does hair grow?
    a. 3 inches per year
    b. 6 inches per year
    c. 8 inches per year
    d. 12 inches per year

22. What is oil that provides protection for the epidermis from external factors and that lubricates both the skin and hair?
    a. lymph
    b. pus
    c. blood
    d. sebum

23. What is the formal name for the horny layer?
    a. stratum corneum
    b. stratum spinosum
    c. stratum granulosum
    d. stratum lucidum

24. What is the technical term for the nail?
    a. onyx
    b. papillae
    c. sebum
    d. lymph

25.   What is true of the stratum corneum?

       a.   It is made of hardened sebum.

       b.   It is the outermost layer of the skin.

       c.   It is the innermost layer of the skin.

       d.   It is devoid of corneocytes.

26.   What happens in the stratum germinativum

       a.   Desmosomes are dissolved.

       b.   Cells divide.

       c.   Cells release lipids, forming bilayers of oil and water.

       d.   Desquamation occurs.

27.   What happens in the stratum granulosum?

       a.   Desmosomes are created.

       b.   Langerhans immune cells protect the body.

       c.   Keratin is produced.

       d.   Fingerprints are formed.

28.   What part of the skin provides a protective cushion and energy storage for the body?

       a.   epidermis

       b.   subcutaneous layer

       c.   dermis

       d.   barrier function

29.   What are the glands that excrete perspiration, regulate body temperature, and detoxify the body?

       a.   sudoriferous

       b.   thyroid

       c.   hyperthyroid

       d.   pituitary

30.   What is telangiectasia?

       a.   capillary wall dilation

       b.   follicle damage

       c.   aging

       d.   poor nutrition

31. What causes transepidermal water loss?
    a. perspiration
    b. evaporation
    c. salivation
    d. secretion

32. What is the dermis?
    a. innermost layer of the skin
    b. outermost layer of the skin
    c. support layer above the epidermis
    d. support layer below the epidermis

33. Which nerves react to heat, cold, pain, pressure, and touch?
    a. motor
    b. secretory
    c. sensory
    d. efferent

34. What protein fiber is found in the dermis and gives skin its flexibility and firmness?
    a. collagen
    b. melanin
    c. keratin
    d. elastin

35. What hormone stimulates cells to reproduce and heal?
    a. dermal stimulant factor (DSF)
    b. epidermal growth factor (EGF)
    c. integumentary regulatory factor (IRF)
    d. integumentary manufacturing factor (IMF)

36. What is true of the epidermis?
    a. It is the outermost layer of the skin.
    b. It is the innermost layer of the skin.
    c. It is below the dermis.
    d. It is below the subcutaneous layer.

37. What comprises about 50 to 70 percent of the skin?
    a. lymph
    b. water
    c. oil
    d. pus

38. What causes the body to produce its own vitamin D?

     a. drinking orange juice

     b. exposure to the sun

     c. drinking a liter of water

     d. exposure to heat

39. What is not one of the six primary functions of the skin?

     a. heat regulation

     b. sensation

     c. absorption

     d. reflection

40. When do free radicals produce more free radicals?

     a. before causing oxidation reactions

     b. while causing oxidation reactions

     c. only when exposed to hydrogen

     d. only when exposed to carbon

41. What function do the sudoriferous glands perform?

     a. assist in holding cells together

     b. excrete perspiration, regulate body temperature, and detoxify the body

     c. stimulate cells to reproduce and heal

     d. stimulate cells, collagen, and amino acids that form proteins

42. Eccrine glands are _____.

     a. taste buds

     b. sweat glands

     c. goose bumps

     d. leukocytes

43. _____ are the basic material and building blocks of the body's tissues.

     a. Proteins

     b. Cells

     c. Glands

     d. Appendages

44. What are sweat glands that are found all over the body with openings on the skin's surface through pores and that are not attached to hair follicles?

    a. apocrine

    b. eccrine

    c. sebaceous

    d. sudoriferous

45. What function do sebaceous glands perform?

    a. protect the surface of the skin

    b. excrete perspiration and regulate body temperature

    c. produce skin pigment granules in the basal layer

    d. stimulate cells, collagen, and amino acids that form proteins

46. Estheticians who specialize in the health and beauty of skin are sometime referred to as _____.

    a. facialists

    b. anatomists

    c. histologists

    d. technicians

47. Estheticians should be able to interpret the effects of which factor that influences skin health and appearance?

    a. hormones

    b. nutrition

    c. ultraviolet damage

    d. all of the above

48. What is an esthetician's primary focus?

    a. preserve the skin

    b. protect the skin

    c. nourish the skin

    d. all of the above

49. What does scar tissue lack?

    a. melanin and elastin

    b. hair and sweat glands

    c. collagen and elastin

    d. hair and melanin

50. Estheticians should have a thorough understanding of the physiology and histology of the skin for all the following reasons EXCEPT to _____.

    a. understand how the skin and the other body parts work together

    b. understand the effects of ultraviolet (UV) damage, hormonal influences, and nutrition on skin health

    c. confidently treat the body to maintain optimum health

    d. be able to help clients choose hormone replacement therapy programs

51. What percentage of hard B-keratin does hair contain?

    a. 50 percent

    b. 75 percent

    c. 90 percent

    d. 20 percent

52. How is B-keratin different from A-keratin?

    a. It breaks more easily than A-keratin.

    b. It has lower moisture and fat than A-keratin.

    c. It is softer than A-keratin.

    d. It flakes away more easily than A-keratin.

53. Which of the following statements is true about the nail plate?

    a. It contains no nerves.

    b. It has many blood vessels.

    c. It is soft and thin.

    d. It is composed of A-keratin.

54. If a person has a purple or bluish tone under their fingernails, then they most likely have which condition?

    a. rosacea

    b. telangiectasia

    c. diabetes

    d. cyanosis

55. Which nerves convey impulses from the brain or spinal cord to the muscles or glands?

    a. motor

    b. secretory

    c. sensory

    d. afferent

CHAPTER 4
DISORDERS AND DISEASES OF THE SKIN

EXPLAIN WHY KNOWLEDGE OF DISEASES AND DISORDERS IS VALUABLE FOR AN ESTHETICIAN

SHORT ANSWER

1. Why should estheticians have a thorough understanding of skin diseases and disorders?

_____

_____

_____

_____

_____

_____

DESCRIBE HOW AN ESTHETICIAN AND A DERMATOLOGIST CAN WORK COLLABORATIVELY

MULTIPLE CHOICE

2. What is the branch of medical science that studies and treats the skin and its disorders?

    a. endocrinology   c. cardiology

    b. dermatology   d. hematology

SHORT ANSWER

3. Since an esthetician cannot diagnose disorders and diseases of the skin, how can they be a partner with a dermatologist?

_____

_____

_____

_____

_____

IDENTIFY THE DIFFERENCE BETWEEN PRIMARY, SECONDARY, AND TERTIARY SKIN LESIONS

SHORT ANSWER

4. What are lesions?

_____

_____

_____

_____

_____

MATCHING

5. Match the three types of lesions with the correct definition.

| a. primary lesion | b. secondary lesion | c. tertiary lesion |

_____ lesions in the initial stages of development or change; characterized by flat, nonpalpable changes in skin color or by elevations formed by fluid in a cavity, such as vesicles or pustules

_____ also known as *vascular lesions*; vascular lesions involve the blood or circulatory system

_____ characterized by piles of material on the skin surface, such as a crust or scab, or by depressions in the skin surface, such as an ulcer; these may require medical referral

Primary and Secondary Skin Lesions

FILL IN THE BLANK

6. Complete the chart on the following page listing P for primary or S for secondary lesions, their characteristics, and whether a salon service can be performed on the client. The first example has been provided for you.

Lesion	Primary or Secondary (P or S)	Description	Does it require a medical referral? (Y or N)
Bulla	P	Large blisters containing watery fluid	N
Cyst/ Tubercle			
Crust			
Excoriation			
Fissure			
Keloid			
Macule			
Nodule			
Papule			
Pustule			
Scale			
Scar/ Cicatrix			
Tumor			
Ulcer			
Vesicle			
Wheal			

RECOGNIZE SKIN CHANGES THAT COULD INDICATE A TYPE OF SKIN CANCER

SHORT ANSWER

7. What causes skin cancer?

_____

_____

_____

_____

_____

Types of Skin Cancer

MATCHING

8. Match the descriptions to the types of cancer. Terms may be used more than once.

a. actinic keratosis	c. squamous cell carcinoma
b. basal cell carcinoma	d. malignant melanoma

_____ most common type of skin cancer

_____ pink or flesh-colored

_____ deadly

_____ cells can grow and spread to other areas of the body

_____ least severe type of skin cancer

_____ can metastasize throughout the body

_____ feels sharp or rough

_____ characterized by scaly, red or pink papules or nodules

ABCDEs of Melanoma Detection

SHORT ANSWER

9. List the skin changes to look for when checking moles.

_____

_____

_____

_____

_____

DESCRIBE THE TYPES OF ACNE

SHORT ANSWER

10. What is acne?

_____

_____

_____

_____

_____

Types of Clogged Follicles

MATCHING

11. Match the descriptions to the types of clogged follicle. Terms may be used more than once.

a. comedo	e. milia
b. open comedo	f. retention hyperkeratosis
c. closed comedo	g. sebaceous hyperplasia
d. sebaceous filaments	h. seborrhea

_____ snags unwanted hair and epilates them

_____ small, solidified impactions of oil without the cell matter

_____ hereditary factor in which dead skin cells build up

_____ a noninflamed buildup of cells, sebum, and other debris inside follicles

_____ whitish, pearl-like masses of sebum

_____ in the scalp it is called dandruff

_____ more common in dry skin types

_____ often white, yellow, or flesh-colored

_____ blackhead open at the surface and exposed to air

_____ forms when the openings of the follicles are blocked with debris

_____ described as doughnut-shaped with an indentation in the center

_____ often found on the nose

_____ applied in soft or hard form

_____ usually found around the eyes, cheeks, and forehead

Grades of Acne

FILL IN THE BLANK

12. Fill in the grade of acne for each description.

Grade	Description
	Red and inflamed; many comedones, papules, and pustules
	Cystic acne; cysts with comedones, papules, pustules, and inflammation; scar formation from tissue damage is common
	Minor breakouts, mostly open comedones, some closed comedones, and a few papules
	Many closed comedones, more open comedones, and occasional papules and pustules

Acne Triggers

MIND MAPPING

13. For each of the acne triggers, describe it and how you would treat it.

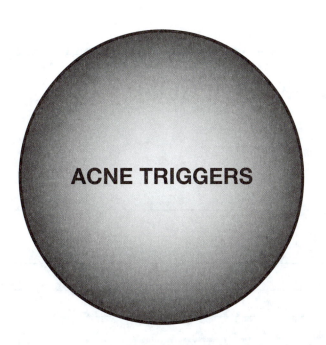

Medicated Treatment Options for Acne

MULTIPLE CHOICE

14. Why are medical professionals reducing the use of antibiotic treatments for acne?

      a. the risk of antibiotic resistance

      b. the cost

      c. the side effects

      d. the availability

15. Antibiotics for acne can be used _____.

      a. only topically

      b. only orally

      c. neither topically or orally

      d. both topically and orally

DESCRIBE THE SYMPTOMS OF POLYCYSTIC OVARIAN SYNDROME (PCOS)

SHORT ANSWER

16. Describe PCOS symptoms.

_____

_____

_____

_____

_____

_____

17. How will an esthetician help a client with PCOS?

_____

_____

_____

_____

_____

_____

LIST COMMON VASCULAR CONDITIONS OR DISORDERS

TRUE OR FALSE

18. For the following statements on vascular conditions or disorders, circle T if true or F if false.

   T   F   Rosacea starts with flushing and increasing bouts of redness.

   T   F   Rosacea cannot affect the eyes.

   T   F   Spicy foods, alcohol, caffeine, temperature extremes, heat, sun, and stress aggravate rosacea symptoms.

   T   F   Provide soothing facials with gentle massage and light exfoliation to treat rosacea.

   T   F   Telangiectasia is visible capillaries commonly found on the face, particularly around the nose, cheeks, and chin.

   T   F   Telangiectasia is a cosmetic irregularity and a medical condition.

   T   F   As a treatment for varicose veins, *sclerotherapy* can cause smaller vessels to disappear.

IDENTIFY PIGMENT DISORDERS

SHORT ANSWER

19. Describe the difference between hyperpigmentation and hypopigmentation.

_____

_____

_____

_____

_____

20. List two causes of pigment disorders.

_____

_____

_____

_____

_____

Hyperpigmentation

COLLAGE

21. Create a collage depicting the different types of hyperpigmentation found on the skin. For each one list its describable characteristics and where it is typically found on the body. You may create your collage in the space below, on a separate sheet of paper, or digitally.

Hypopigmentation

FILL IN THE BLANK

22. Fill in the blank for the types of hypopigmentation disorders.

_____ is a loss of pigmentation leading to light, abnormal patches of depigmented skin. It is a congenital disorder acquired due to immunological and post-inflammatory causes.

_____ is a rare genetic condition characterized by a lack of melanin pigment in the body, including the skin, hair, and eyes. The person is at risk for skin cancer, is sensitive to light, and ages early without normal melanin protection.

_____ is a pigmentation disease characterized by irregular white patches of skin that are totally lacking pigment. The condition can worsen with time and exposure to sunlight. The disease can occur at any age and is believed to be an autoimmune disorder causing an absence of melanocytes.

SHORT ANSWER

23. How is tinea versicolor different than the other hypopigmentation disorders?

_____

_____

_____

_____

_____

_____

DESCRIBE THE DIFFERENT TYPES OF DERMATITIS

SHORT ANSWER

24. What is dermatitis?

_____

_____

_____

_____

_____

FILL IN THE BLANK

25. Complete the following statements about the types of dermatitis.

Occupational disorders from ingredients in cosmetics and chemical solutions can cause

_____.

_____ is caused by exposure to and direct skin contact with an allergen.

_____ is an increased or exaggerated sensitivity to products.

Topical corticosteroids can relieve the symptoms of _____.

An inflammatory, painful itching disease of the skin that can be acute or chronic in nature with dry or moist lesions is _____.

_____ are examples of irritants that can cause _____.

When the skin is damaged by irritating substances, the immune system springs into action, flooding the tissue with water, which causes _____.

_____ is an acne-like condition around the mouth that may be caused by toothpaste or products used on the face.

The red, flaky skin of _____ _____ often appears in the eyebrows, on the scalp and along the hairline, in the middle of the forehead, and along the sides of the nose.

_____ is caused by poor circulation in the lower legs and can create a chronic inflammatory state.

IDENTIFY THE TYPES OF HYPERTROPHIES

SHORT ANSWER

26. List and describe the types of hypertrophies.

_____

_____

_____

_____

_____

_____

_____

_____

_____

_____

_____

_____

_____

_____

_____

_____

_____

_____

_____

_____

_____

_____

DEFINE NINE CONTAGIOUS SKIN AND NAIL DISEASES

MATCHING

27. Match the descriptions of the nine contagious skin and nail diseases to the terms.

a. conjunctivitis	d. herpes zoster	g. tinea
b. herpes simplex virus 1	e. impetigo	h. tinea corporis
c. herpes simplex virus 2	f. onychomycosis	i. verruca

_____ clusters of small blisters or crusty lesions

_____ pinkeye

_____ ringworm

_____ shingles

_____ fever blisters or cold sores

_____ wart

_____ fungal infection

_____ peels, waxing, or other stimuli may cause a breakout

_____ thick, brittle, discolored nails

IDENTIFY TWO MENTAL HEALTH CONDITIONS THAT MAY MANIFEST AS SKIN CONDITIONS

SHORT ANSWER

28. Describe the two mental health conditions you may encounter as an esthetician.

_____

_____

_____

_____

_____

RECOGNIZE COMMON SKIN CONDITIONS RELATED TO SKIN DISEASES AND DISORDERS

TRUE OR FALSE

29. For the following statements on skin conditions, circle T if true or F if false.

T F   A furuncle is also known as a boil.

T F   A group of boils is called an edema.

T F   Swelling from a fluid imbalance is a carbuncle.

T F   Erythema is redness caused by inflammation.

T F   When hair grows under the surface of the skin instead of growing up and out of the follicle, causing a bacterial infection, it is called folliculitis.

T F   Razor bumps are the common name for pruritus.

T F   The medical term for persistent itching is _steatoma_.

T F   A sebaceous cyst filled with sebum is called pseudofolliculitis.

EXPLAIN FIVE SUDORIFEROUS GLAND DISORDERS

SHORT ANSWER

30. Explain the five sudoriferous gland disorders.

• _____

_____

• _____

_____

- _____
  _____
- _____
  _____
- _____
  _____

SHORT ANSWER

31. How will knowing about disorders and diseases of the skin help you as an esthetician?

_____
_____
_____
_____
_____

WORD REVIEW

MULTIPLE CHOICE

32. The medical term for hives is _____.

   a. folliculitis

   b. erythema

   c. urticaria

   d. perioral dermatitis

33. A cyst may contain _____.

   a. fluid

   b. infection

   c. other matter above or below the skin

   d. all of the above

34. Scratching or scraping the skin can produce a(n) _____.

   a. excoriation

   b. fissure

   c. keloid

   d. ulcer

35. A thin plate of epidermal cells is called _____.

   a. dry skin

   b. dandruff

   c. asteatosis

   d. scale

36. When tissue hardens to heal an injury, it results in a(n) _____.

   a. crust

   b. scar

   c. cyst

   d. excoriation

37. Which of these conditions often appears as light, pearly nodules?

   a. basal cell carcinoma

   b. malignant melanoma

   c. herpes simplex

   d. bacterial conjunctivitis

38. The second most serious form of skin cancer is _____.

  a. malignant melanoma

  b. malignant carcinoma

  c. basal cell carcinoma

  d. squamous cell carcinoma

39. What is the most deadly form of skin cancer?

  a. squamous cell carcinoma

  b. malignant melanoma

  c. basal cell carcinoma

  d. squamous-basal carcinoma

40. What are nodules?

  a. brown or wine-colored discolorations

  b. small bumps caused by conditions such as scar tissue or infections

  c. large blisters containing watery fluid

  d. clusters of boils

41. What is a tubercle?

  a. open lesion on the skin or mucous membrane of the body

  b. abnormal rounded, solid lump larger than a papule

  c. yeast infection of the skin that inhibits melanin production

  d. another name for the contagious infection called ringworm

42. What is a characteristic of the form of skin cancer called squamous cell carcinoma?

  a. pearly translucency to fleshy color

  b. dark purple splotches at the joints

  c. scaly red or pink papules or nodules

  d. asymmetrical area and color variation

43. What is a light-colored, slightly raised mark on the skin that is formed after an injury or lesion of the skin has healed?

  a. stain

  b. wheal

  c. tan

  d. scar

44.   What is a bulla?

    a.   mass of hardened sebum and skin cells in a hair follicle

    b.   open comedone

    c.   closed comedone

    d.   large blister containing watery fluid that is larger than a vesicle

45.   What is a thick scar resulting from excessive growth of fibrous tissue (collagen)?

    a.   stain

    b.   keloid

    c.   wheal

    d.   wen

46.   What are secondary lesions?

    a.   benign outgrowths of the skin that look like flaps

    b.   thick scars resulting from excessive growth of fibrous tissue

    c.   brown or wine-colored discolorations

    d.   skin damage that changes the structure of tissues or organs

47.   What is a pustule?

    a.   irritated vesicle

    b.   inflamed papule

    c.   inflamed wheal

    d.   irritated wen

48.   What is true of a comedogenic product?

    a.   It tends to clog follicles and cause a buildup of dead skin cells.

    b.   It has no adverse effects on the skin whatsoever.

    c.   It helps clear up comedones quickly and safely.

    d.   This sort of product should not be used on human skin.

49.   What is crust an accumulation of?

    a.   sweat and dirt

    b.   water and salt

    c.   sebum and pus

    d.   blood and lymph

50.   What are not examples of wheals?

    a.   hives

    b.   mosquito bites

    c.   urticaria

    d.   pustules

51.   What is a small blister or sac containing clear fluid called?

    a.   vesicle

    b.   carbuncle

    c.   melanoma

    d.   wen

52.   What is the common name for urticaria, which is caused by an allergic reaction from the body's production of histamine?

    a.   pinkeye

    b.   ringworm

    c.   scabies

    d.   hives

53.   What accompanies an ulcer in addition to a loss of skin depth?

    a.   pus

    b.   blood

    c.   lymph

    d.   sebum

54.   What is the term for an abnormal cell mass that results from excessive cell multiplication and varies in size, shape, and color?

    a.   tumor

    b.   comedone

    c.   skin tag

    d.   razor bump

DISCOVERIES AND ACCOMPLISHMENTS

In the space below, write notes about key concepts discussed in this chapter. Share your discoveries with some of the other students in your class and ask them if your notes are helpful. You may want to revise your discoveries based on good ideas shared by your peers.

Discoveries:

_____

_____

_____

_____

_____

_____

_____

_____

_____

_____

List at least three things you have accomplished since your last entry that relate to learning skin disorders and diseases.

Accomplishments:

_____

_____

_____

_____

_____

_____

_____

_____

EXAM REVIEW

MULTIPLE CHOICE

1. What term is used to describe any mark, wound, or abnormality?

    a. lesion

    b. papule

    c. cyst

    d. skin tag

2. What is leukoderma?

    a. flat, hairy spots on the skin

    b. light, abnormal patches of depigmented skin

    c. brown or wine-colored discoloration

    d. thick scar resulting from excessive fibrous tissue

3. What is the term for a flat spot or discoloration of the skin, such as a freckle?

    a. pustule

    b. cyst

    c. macule

    d. stain

4. What is true of malignant melanoma?

    a. It is a benign form of skin cancer.

    b. It is the least serious form of skin cancer.

    c. It is a moderately serious form of skin cancer.

    d. It is the most serious form of skin cancer.

5. What condition is also known as melasma?

    a. hyperpigmentation

    b. hypopigmentation

    c. benign melanoma

    d. malignant melanoma

6. What is an example of epidermal cysts?

    a. scars

    b. milia

    c. boils

    d. blisters

7. What is another name for the acute inflammatory disorder miliaria rubra?

    a. prickly heat

    b. scabies

    c. rabies

    d. shingles

8. What term refers to a pigmented nevus?

    a. nodule

    b. vesicle

    c. papule

    d. mole

9. What is another name for a nevus?

    a. carbuncle

    b. wheal

    c. birthmark

    d. skin tag

10. What is tinea versicolor?

    a. pigmentation disease characterized by white patches

    b. yeast infection of the skin that inhibits melanin production

    c. generic term for any kind of fungal infection

    d. severe oiliness of the skin

11. What is the common name for the contagious infection tinea corporis?

    a. ringworm

    b. shingles

    c. rabies

    d. scabies

12. What is the generic term for a fungal infection?

    a. miliaria

    b. tinea

    c. verruca

    d. barbae

13. What is the scientific term for couperose skin?

    a. tinea barbae

    b. tinea pedis

    c. telangiectasia

    d. pseudofolliculitis

14. What is a steatoma?

    a. brown or wine-colored discoloration

    b. sebaceous cyst of subcutaneous tumor filled with sebum

    c. brownish spot ranging in color from tan to bluish-black

    d. small, benign outgrowth of the skin that looks like a flap

15. What is the term for a brown or wine-colored discoloration?

    a. wen

    b. wheal

    c. tan

    d. stain

16. What are skin tags?

    a. small, benign outgrowths of the skin that look like flaps

    b. dangerous manifestations of malignant melanoma

    c. thick scars resulting from excessive fibrous tissue

    d. decaying discharges from infected comedones

17. What is rosacea?

    a. any skin with a naturally rose-hued color

    b. condition characterized by redness and dilation of blood vessels

    c. light-colored, raised mark on the skin formed after injury

    d. skin cream used for treating fair-skinned clients

18. What are sebaceous filaments?

    a. mainly solidified impactions of oil without the cell matter

    b. light-colored, slightly raised marks on the skin formed after injuries

    c. thin plates of epidermal flakes, such as excessive dandruff

    d. small clusters of papules caused by products used on the face

19.   What is an example of sebaceous hyperplasia?

    a.   benign lesions frequently seen in oilier areas of the face

    b.   solidified impactions of oil without the cell matter

    c.   light-colored, slightly raised marks on the skin formed after injuries

    d.   patches covered with white-silver scales

20.   What is acne?

    a.   medical condition defined by an absence of melanin pigment

    b.   chronic inflammatory skin disorder of the sebaceous glands

    c.   excess inflammation from allergies and irritants

    d.   foul-smelling perspiration, usually in the armpits or feet

21.   What are actinic keratoses?

    a.   large blisters containing watery fluid that are similar to vesicles

    b.   clusters of boils

    c.   pink or flesh-colored precancerous lesions that result from sun damage

    d.   closed, abnormally developed sacs

22.   What is albinism?

    a.   deficiency in perspiration

    b.   dry, scaly skin resulting from sebum deficiency

    c.   foul-smelling perspiration

    d.   medical condition defined by an absence of melanin pigment

23.   What is anhidrosis?

    a.   deficiency in perspiration

    b.   excessive perspiration

    c.   foul-smelling perspiration

    d.   bloody perspiration

24.   What is the term for excess inflammation (dry skin, redness, itching) from allergies and irritants?

    a.   squamous cell melanoma

    b.   contact dermatitis

    c.   atopic dermatitis

    d.   basal cell melanoma

25. What is true of basal cell carcinoma?
    a. It is the least common type of skin cancer.
    b. It is the least severe type of skin cancer.
    c. It is the most serious type of skin cancer.
    d. It is a benign form of skin cancer.

26. What is the term for foul-smelling perspiration, usually in the armpits or on the feet?
    a. tinea pedis
    b. bromhidrosis
    c. asteatosis
    d. tinea barbae

27. What is hyperkeratosis?
    a. overproduction of pigment
    b. underproduction of pigment
    c. thickening of the skin caused by a mass of keratinized cells
    d. thinning of the skin caused by a lack of keratinized cells

28. What is the term for the overproduction of pigment?
    a. hyperpigmentation
    b. superpigmentation
    c. metapigmentation
    d. hypopigmentation

29. What is hypertrophy?
    a. abnormal growth
    b. normal growth
    c. abnormal perspiration
    d. normal perspiration

30. What is hypopigmentation?
    a. excess of pigment
    b. injection of pigment
    c. surgical removal of pigment
    d. lack of pigment

31. What is impetigo?

      a. light, abnormal patches that are the result of congenital defects

      b. scar tissue resulting from excessive growth of fibrous tissue

      c. contagious bacterial infection marked by clusters of small blisters

      d. redness and bumpiness in the cheeks caused by blocked follicles

32. What is a keratoma?

      a. thick scar resulting from excessive growth of fibrous tissue

      b. open comedone

      c. closed comedone

      d. acquired, thickened patch of epidermis

33. What is keratosis pilaris?

      a. acquired, thickened patch of epidermis

      b. redness and bumpiness in the cheeks caused by blocked follicles

      c. most malignant form of skin cancer

      d. least malignant form of skin cancer

34. Where in the face does the acne-like condition perioral dermatitis manifest?

      a. forehead

      b. chin

      c. nose

      d. mouth

35. What is a characteristic of primary lesions?

      a. brownish spots ranging in color from tan to bluish-black

      b. subcutaneous tumors filled with sebum

      c. infection with ringed, red pattern with elevated ridges

      d. flat, nonpalpable changes in skin color

36. When someone has retention hyperkeratosis, what builds up and fails to shed from the follicles as happens in normal skin?

      a. sebum

      b. dead skin cells

      c. perspiration

      d. hairs

37. What is the common name for the very contagious infection conjunctivitis?

      a. ringworm

      b. pinkeye

      c. rabies

      d. scabies

38. What is contact dermatitis?

      a. foul-smelling perspiration

      b. the effect when two skin disorders connect with each other

      c. an inflammation caused by contact with a substance or chemical

      d. excessive perspiration

39. What type of physician specializes in treating skin disorders and diseases?

      a. dermatologist

      b. physiologist

      c. esthetician

      d. cosmetologist

40. What is vitiligo?

      a. contagious skin condition

      b. allergic reaction to strong chemicals in cleaning products

      c. total absence of pigmentation

      d. pigmentation disease characterized by white patches

41. What is the common name for the hypertrophy of the papillae and epidermis known as a verruca?

      a. wheal

      b. wart

      c. wen

      d. wick

42. What is eczema?

      a. pigmentation disease characterized by white patches

      b. inflammatory, painful itching disease of the skin

      c. yeast infection on the skin that inhibits melanin production

      d. contagious infection that forms a ringed, red pattern

43. What is edema?

      a. any inflammatory condition of the skin

      b. swelling caused by a fluid imbalance in cells

      c. brownish spot ranging in color from tan to bluish-black

      d. closed, abnormally developed sac containing fluid or other matter

44. What is erythema?

      a. oiliness caused by inflammation

      b. redness caused by inflammation

      c. dryness caused by inflammation

      d. pain caused by inflammation

45. What is true of herpes simplex virus 1?

      a. It causes fever blisters and cold sores.

      b. It causes hepatitis.

      c. It is the virus that causes AIDS.

      d. It is always a terminal condition.

46. What is hyperhidrosis?

      a. insufficient perspiration

      b. excessive perspiration

      c. foul-smelling perspiration

      d. sweet-smelling perspiration

47. When you do not recognize a skin condition, what should you do?

      a. post a photo on social media asking others for advice

      b. stop the service and diagnose the problem

      c. continue to provide the service, since that is your job

      d. stop the service and refer the client to their doctor

48. Which of the following statements about PCOS is true?

      a. It is not a condition that is cured, but it can be managed.

      b. It is not a condition that is cured, nor can it be managed.

      c. It is a condition that can be cured if managed well.

      d. It is a condition that can be cured with little to no management.

49. What mental health condition may cause the client to become a spa hopper, because they are never satisfied with their appearance?

    a. poikiloderma of Civatte

    b. body dysmorphic disorder

    c. dermatillomania

    d. onychomycosis

50. By recognizing a potentially contagious skin disorder, you can _____.

    a. diagnose a treatment

    b. be selective with your clientele

    c. refuse services

    d. stop the spread of infection

51. What is the least severe type of skin cancer?

    a. basal cell carcinoma

    b. melanoma

    c. squamous cell carcinoma

    d. melasma

52. What do the letters ABCDE stand for in regard to the ABCDE Cancer Checklist?

    a. asymmetrical, borders, color, diameter, evolve

    b. abnormal, borders, color, diagnose, expose

    c. asymmetrical, basal, carcinoma, diameter, eradicate

    d. abnormal, borders, carcinoma, diagnose, eradicate

53. Dionne tells Tyree that she has a condition known as prickly heat. Tyree thinks Dionne may have used the wrong name for her condition because prickly heat, also known as _____, is characterized by the appearance of red vesicles and burning, itchy skin upon exposure to excessive heat.

    a. hyperhidrosis

    b. miliaria rubra

    c. anhidrosis

    d. bromhidrosis

54. Recently, Tori noticed some patches of red, itchy skin on her face, and she made an appointment with her dermatologist and confirmed she could continue to go for facial or skin treatments. She makes an appointment with her esthetician, Kris, a few weeks later and has since forgotten what the condition was called. Tori thinks back and says the condition must be _____. Kris disagrees, since this condition is characterized by extreme redness, dilation of blood vessels, and in severe cases, the formation of papules and pustules.

    a. telangiectasia

    b. rosacea

    c. edema

    d. varicose veins

55.   What is the term for dilated and twisted veins?

    a.   varicose veins

    b.   vesicle veins

    c.   verruca veins

    d.   vitiligo veins

56.   What is the most common cancer diagnosis for men over age 50?

    a.   colon cancer

    b.   lung cancer

    c.   prostate cancer

    d.   skin cancer

57.   If you had one bad sunburn in childhood, what is true of your risk for melanoma later in life?

    a.   It is quadrupled.

    b.   It is tripled.

    c.   It is doubled.

    d.   It remains the same.

58.   What is the skin disease characterized by red patches covered with white-silver scales?

    a.   psoriasis

    b.   eczema

    c.   rosacea

    d.   melasma

59.   Which of the following gives the appearance of "chicken skin"?

    a.   keratosis

    b.   keratosis pilaris

    c.   hyperkeratosis

    d.   psoriasis

60.   Women experiencing menopause may also experience which of the following conditions?

    a.   hyperhidrosis

    b.   bromhidrosis

    c.   anhidrosis

    d.   diaphoresis

CHAPTER 5
SKIN ANALYSIS

EXPLAIN THE PROCESS OF SKIN ANALYSIS

SHORT ANSWER

1. Why should estheticians study skin analysis?

_____

_____

_____

_____

_____

_____

IDENTIFY THE FOUR GENETIC SKIN TYPES THROUGH VISUALIZATION, PALPATION, AND CONSULTATION

TRUE OR FALSE

2. Circle whether the following statements are true or false.

   T F   Only three of the skin types need proper cleansing, exfoliating, hydrating, and protecting.

   T F   Estheticians use consultation to determine conditions of the skin, like oiliness and hydration.

   T F   Evaluating pores in the T-zone is the first step in determining skin type.

   T F   Skin analysis uses visualization to note skin properties, like pore size and blemishes.

   T F   Skin type is determined by the reaction of skin to UV radiation.

MATCHING

3. Match the characteristic to the skin type. Choices may be used more than once.

a. normal	c. oily
b. combination	d. dry

_____ very small follicle size

_____ shiny appearance

_____ flaky and blotchy

_____ hydrated to dehydrated

_____ tight

_____ good elasticity

_____ thick and firm

_____ oilier in t-zone

4. Match the treatment to the skin type. Choices may be used more than once.

a. normal	c. oily
b. combination	d. dry

_____ treatments to balance oil production

_____ maintenance and protection treatments

_____ treatments using oil-based products

_____ regular cleansing and exfoliation, and hydrating with water-based products

_____ treatments to provide nourishment and protection

_____ avoid harsh products and rough exfoliation

DIFFERENTIATE THE SIX FITZPATRICK SKIN TYPES AND ACCURATELY IDENTIFY THEM

COLLAGE

5. Using photos from magazines, websites, or your personal collection, assemble a collage for each of the different Fitzpatrick skin types. You may create your collage on a separate sheet of paper or digitally.

DISTINGUISH THE CHARACTERISTICS OF SENSITIVE SKIN

MULTIPLE CHOICE

6. Which of the following are characteristics of sensitive skin?

    a. difficult to wax, oily, and irritated by the sun

    b. dehydrated, large comedones, and redness

    c. fragility, thin skin, and redness

    d. oily, hyperpigmented, and thick skin

7. Clients with which Fitzpatrick skin type tend to have more sensitive skin?

    a. skin type I

    b. skin type V

    c. skin type VI

    d. skin type III

8. Sensitive skin can become irritated by what stimulation?

    a. heat

    b. exfoliation

    c. extractions

    d. all of the above

RECOGNIZE THE INTRICACIES INVOLVED WITH TREATING SKIN OF COLOR

TRUE OR FALSE

9. For the following statements on treating skin of color, circle T if true or F if false.

   T F   Type IV is considered to be one of the least challenging skin types to treat well.

   T F   Fitzpatrick skin type IV does not show signs of aging as quickly as types I and II.

   T F   Fitzpatrick skin types V and VI generally have drier and thinner skin than types I and II.

   T F   When treating skin of color, waxing is easier due to thicker hair and thicker roots in the follicle.

   T F   Darker skin types have melanocytes that produce more melanin than light skin types.

IDENTIFY TREATMENT OPTIONS FOR THE NECK AND DÉCOLLETÉ

FILL IN THE BLANK

10. Tech neck, a new phenomenon caused by the repeated movement of looking down at a cell phone or other electronic device, has created a demand for specialty topical treatments that include

_____, _____, and _____.

11. The neck and décolleté show aging more quickly because they have fewer _____ glands than the face.

12. _____ and _____ products may cause excess irritation to the area.

ILLUSTRATE EXAMPLES OF SKIN CONDITIONS VERSUS SKIN TYPES

COLLAGE

13. Using photos from magazines, websites, or your personal collection, assemble a collage depicting and labeling your skin type, two of your friends' skin types, and three different skin conditions. You may create your collage on a separate sheet of paper or digitally.

EXPLAIN THE CAUSES OF SKIN CONDITIONS

SHORT ANSWER

14. Why is it important as an esthetician to understand factors that affect the skin?

_____

_____

_____

_____

_____

External Factors that Affect the Skin

SHORT ANSWER

15. List four external factors that can affect the skin.

_____

_____

_____

_____

_____

_____

_____

_____

_____

_____

_____

Internal Factors that Affect the Skin

SHORT ANSWER

16. Name three internal factors that are affecting your skin.

_____

_____

_____

_____

_____

_____

_____

_____

_____

_____

DESCRIBE HEALTHY HABITS FOR THE SKIN

ESSAY

17. How will you encourage your clients to practice healthy habits for better skin?

_____

_____

_____

_____

_____

_____

_____

_____

_____

_____

_____

DETERMINE TREATMENT CONTRAINDICATIONS THROUGH EVALUATION, ANAYLSIS, AND CONSULTATION

MULTIPLE CHOICE

18. Which of the following would not cause a contraindication with a skin product?

    a. medication

    b. skin color

    c. communicable disease

    d. medical condition

19. Which of the following is a contraindication for waxing treatments?

    a. a pacemaker

    b. blood thinners

    c. pregnancy

    d. metal bone pins or plates in the body

20. A client has just started using an exfoliating topical medication. What treatment are you able to perform?

       a. exfoliation

       b. waxing

       c. electrical

       d. peeling

Client Consultations

MULTIPLE CHOICE

21. What is the most important reason to complete a client consultation?

       a. to determine why a client is happy

       b. to sell the client on additional treatments

       c. to build a better relationship with your client

       d. to determine whether a treatment is appropriate for the client

SHORT ANSWER

22. Create a list of questions you will ask yourself in preparation for a client consultation.

_____

_____

_____

_____

_____

23. Describe the three forms you will use with a new client.

- _____

  _____

- _____

  _____

- _____

  _____

FILL IN THE BLANK

24. A client has scheduled their first appointment. You should ask them to come in _____ before their appointment time to complete the client intake form.

25. After reviewing the treatment process and the client signs the consent form, _____ and keep original for your files.

Case Study

26. You will have a new client tomorrow. You know from the client, when she called to schedule, that she is new to the area, about 35 years old, and does not use any special products, just Bath and Body Works lotions. Write down the questions you will ask during the consultation.

_____

_____

_____

_____

_____

_____

_____

_____

_____

_____

PERFORM A SKIN ANALYSIS

ESSAY

27. Describe how you will perform a skin analysis.

_____

_____

_____

_____

_____

_____

_____

_____

_____

WORD REVIEW

MATCHING

28. Match the term to the correct definition.

a. glycation	i. photosensitivity
b. genetic	j. skin type
c. hypertrichosis	k. "tech neck"
d. palpation	l. contraindications
e. Wood's lamp	m. Fitzpatrick scale
f. dehydration	n. melasma
g. couperose	o. T-zone
h. décolleté	

_____ manual manipulation of tissue by touching to make an assessment of it condition

_____ pertaining to a woman's lower neck and chest

_____ classification that describes a person's genetic skin type

_____ filtered black light that is used to illuminate skin disorders

_____ condition of abnormal growth of hair

_____ wrinkles that develop due to repeated motion of looking down at a phone

_____ center area of the face; corresponds to shape formed by forehead, nose, and chin

_____ related to heredity and ancestry of origin

_____ high sensitivity of the skin to UV light

_____ scale used to measure the skin's reaction to the sun

_____ lack of water

_____ distended capillaries from weakening of the capillary walls

_____ caused by an elevation in blood sugar

_____ form of hyperpigmentation characterized by bilateral brown patches

_____ factors that prohibit treatment due to a condition

DISCOVERIES AND ACCOMPLISHMENTS

In the space below, write notes about key concepts discussed in this chapter. Share your discoveries with some of the other students in your class and ask them if your notes are helpful. You may want to revise your discoveries based on good ideas shared by your peers.

Discoveries:

_____

_____

_____

_____

_____

_____

_____

_____

_____

_____

_____

_____

List at least three things you have accomplished since your last entry that relate to skin analysis.

Accomplishments:

_____

_____

_____

_____

_____

_____

_____

_____

_____

_____

_____

EXAM REVIEW

MULTIPLE CHOICE

1. What is a characteristic of seborrhea?

    a. flaking skin

    b. excess hair growth

    c. blisters

    d. wrinkles

2. Which factors that affect the skin are considered intrinsic?

    a. tanning beds

    b. dehydration

    c. allergies

    d. all of the above

3. How would you define these effects on the skin: pollutants, overexfoliation, climate, and photosensitivity?

    a. intrinsic factors

    b. extrinsic factors

    c. circulatory health factors

    d. genetic health factors

4. What is true of sun damage?

    a. It is a myth that sun exposure damages the skin.

    b. Sun damage is only a minor factor in the overall health of the skin.

    c. It is the main intrinsic cause of aging.

    d. It is the main external cause of aging.

5. What does dehydrated skin lack?

    a. oil

    b. water

    c. lymph

    d. sebum

6. What is true of normal skin?

    a. It has a good oil–water balance.

    b. It is very oily.

    c. It lacks luminosity.

    d. The follicles are large.

7. What skin type is associated with the treatment goals of maintenance and preventative care?

    a. combination

    b. dry

    c. normal

    d. oily

8. If your primary treatment goals are to soothe, calm, and protect, then your client most likely has _____ skin.

    a. dry

    b. normal

    c. oily

    d. sensitive

9. Which habit is not healthy for the skin?

    a. plenty of sun exposure

    b. staying hydrated

    c. exercising regularly

    d. none of the above

10. What are contraindications?

    a. instructions for the use of products

    b. instructions for the use of tools

    c. factors that prohibit a treatment

    d. factors that indicate a treatment will be beneficial

11. What type of skin condition is indicated by redness and is the result of distended capillaries from weakening of the capillary walls?

    a. dehydrated skin

    b. asphyxiated skin

    c. striated skin

    d. couperose skin

12. What does the Fitzpatrick scale measure?

    a. skin's ability to tolerate ultraviolet (UV) exposure

    b. skin's ability to tolerate water exposure

    c. skin's ability to absorb products applied to the epidermis

    d. skin's ability to recover from injection punctures

13. When should you analyze the client's skin type and conditions?

    a. before performing services

    b. while performing services

    c. while selecting products

    d. while scheduling the client's next appointment

14. What type on the Fitzpatrick scale is a person with Latin American heritage, dark hair, dark brown eyes, and who rarely burns?

    a. type II

    b. type III

    c. type IV

    d. type V

15. What are the general characteristics of type II skin on the Fitzpatrick scale?

    a. fair-skinned; brown eyes; dark hair; tans wells and burns moderately

    b. very white skin; blond or red hair; light colored eyes; freckles common; always burns and never tans

    c. light skin; varied eye color; varied hair color; burns easily and tans minimally

    d. Mediterranean, Asian, or Hispanic heritage; dark brown hair; tans easily, rarely burns

16. How would you describe the unexposed skin for type VI skin on the Fitzpatrick scale?

    a. almost translucent skin

    b. fair skin

    c. light brown skin

    d. dark brown or black skin

17. What is true of type I skin on the Fitzpatrick scale?

    a. always burns

    b. often burns

    c. sometimes burns

    d. never burns

18. What is true of type VI skin on the Fitzpatrick scale?

    a. always burns

    b. often burns

    c. sometimes burns

    d. may never burn

19. What is a new phenomenon caused by consistently looking down at your cell phone?

    a. rhytides

    b. photodamage

    c. tech neck

    d. décolleté

20. What makes one person's skin darker than another person's skin?

    a. greater amounts of melanin

    b. lesser amounts of melanin

    c. greater amounts of melanocytes

    d. lesser amounts of melanocytes

21. What skin type is more likely to have a greater problem with hyperpigmentation than the other skin types?

      a. pale

      b. fair

      c. medium

      d. dark

22. What is a characteristic of actinic keratosis?

      a. oily patch that does not abate after thorough cleansing

      b. rough area resulting from sun exposure, sometimes peeling off

      c. cluster of comedones surrounded by a field of redness

      d. irritated area exuding pus through cracks in the skin

23. What is a characteristic of erythema?

      a. irregular heartbeat

      b. irregular respiration

      c. redness caused by inflammation

      d. pain caused by swelling

24. Seizures or epilepsy are a contraindication for which treatment?

      a. waxing

      b. chemical peels

      c. electrical and light-based treatments that pulsate

      d. treatments using salicylic acid

25. What are skin types?

      a. medical terms differentiating the oil–water balance of skin

      b. esthetician terms used to identify common skin conditions

      c. classifications that describe a person's genetic skin attributes

      d. pharmaceutical terms referring to thickness of the skin

26. What are skin types primarily based on?

      a. oil production and lipids between cells

      b. skin color

      c. skin reaction to UV exposure

      d. amount of collagen and elastin

27. What can be indicated by the size of the pores in the T-zone and throughout the face?

      a. skin type

      b. blood pressure

      c. internal body temperature

      d. overall health

28. What is not one of the four skin types?

    a. combination

    b. dry

    c. sensitive

    d. oily

29. What skin types require proper cleansing, exfoliating, and hydrating?

    a. normal and oily

    b. dry and oily

    c. normal and combination

    d. all skin types

30. What is a characteristic of dry skin?

    a. tight feeling, slightly rough

    b. loose feeling, soft to the touch

    c. large, spread-out follicles

    d. large, sebum-filled follicles

31. Which internal effect on the skin alters protein structures and decreases biological activity?

    a. free radicals

    b. vitamin deficiencies

    c. hormones

    d. glycation

32. What is a characteristic of oily skin?

    a. extremely small follicles throughout the face

    b. follicles that are visible or larger over most of the face

    c. follicles that are large only on the chin

    d. follicles that are large only on the cheeks

33. What is true of individuals with Fitzpatrick skin type IV?

    a. They can become hyperpigmented from treatments.

    b. They are more likely to have sensitive skin.

    c. Due to their darker skin, their blemishes are harder to see.

    d. They are prone to a form of hyperkeratosis.

34. What helps to keep your skin healthy?

    a. eating a balanced diet

    b. maintaining a calm attitude

    c. getting professional skin care treatments

    d. all of the above

35. What type of skin ages more slowly than the other types?

    a. dry skin

    b. oily skin

    c. normal

    d. sensitive

36. What is a characteristic of sensitive skin?

    a. easy absorption of product

    b. small follicles and dehydrated skin

    c. fragile, thin skin and redness

    d. multiple blemishes

37. What type of skin can be difficult to treat because of its low tolerance for products and stimulation?

    a. oily

    b. combination

    c. normal

    d. sensitive

38. What type on the Fitzpatrick scale is a person with almost translucent skin, blond or red hair, light-colored eyes, and possibly freckles?

    a. type I

    b. type II

    c. type III

    d. type IV

39. What makes the skin of the neck and décolleté different from the skin on the face?

    a. has fewer sebaceous glands

    b. ages more slowly

    c. is less susceptible to irritation

    d. is unaffected by broken capillaries

40. What is it called when you examine skin through touch to determine oiliness and elasticity?

    a. consultation

    b. palpation

    c. hydration evaluation

    d. pore analysis

41. What type of approach will help you to identify healthy habits and behaviors that are detrimental to skin health and allow you to better help your clients?

    a. specialized

    b. passive

    c. direct

    d. holistic

42. Someone who lives along the equator will have a greater number of what compared to someone who lives at the North Pole?

    a. active oil glands

    b. active melanocytes

    c. follicles

    d. comedones

43. What is true of Fitzpatrick skin types V and VI?

    a. need more exfoliation and deep pore cleansing

    b. are considered one of the most challenging skin types to treat well

    c. do not need sun protection

    d. reactions are most apparent on these skin types

44. Where is the décolleté?

    a. behind the ears

    b. under the chin

    c. under the eyes

    d. lower neck and chest

45. What type of products should not be used on the neck, as they may cause irritation?

    a. antioxidants

    b. growth factor serums

    c. alpha hydroxy acids

    d. additional moisturizers

46. What can you do to maintain the results of your home care regimen and more effectively treat the signs of aging?

    a. have a glass of red wine daily

    b. get professional skin care treatments

    c. sun bathe frequently

    d. exercise less to prevent dehydration

47. If your pregnant client does not have written permission from their medical provider, which of the following treatments could you perform?

    a.   chemical peels

    b.   electrical treatment

    c.   treatments with aggressive cleansing

    d.   none of the above

48. If your client is allergic to aspirin, then you should not use products derived from
_____.

    a.   honey

    b.   the mignonette tree

    c.   henna

    d.   willow bark

49. Which form discloses the client's health history, all products and medications, medical conditions, any known allergies or sensitivities, their at-home skin care program, and skin care treatments the client has recently received?

    a.   intake form

    b.   consent form

    c.   service record chart

    d.   post-service questionnaire

50. What should be on the consent form?

    a.   home care recommendation

    b.   products used in treatment

    c.   client's signature

    d.   date for next appointment

51. What is the best tool to analyze the skin?

    a.   lancet

    b.   esthetician's fingers

    c.   magnifying lamp/light

    d.   blotting paper

PROCEDURE 5–1: PERFORMING A SKIN ANALYSIS

Evaluate your practical skills.

CRITERIA	COMPETENT	NEEDS WORK	IMPROVEMENT PLAN
1. Review the client's health history questionnaire. Look for medical conditions, medications, allergies, or other indications that the client is not an appropriate candidate for treatment. While you are reviewing the documentation, ask your client questions for clarification, if necessary.			
2. Wash your hands as instructed in *Milady Standard Foundations*, Procedure 5–1: Proper Handwashing.			
3. Look briefly at your client's skin (including the neck and chest) with your naked eye or a magnifying light. In order to achieve a more accurate analysis you will need to remove your client's makeup in the following step.			
4. Cleanse the skin (a client's normal state of dryness or oiliness may not be as visible immediately after cleansing).			
5. Cover the eyes with eye pads. Make sure the eye pads are not too large or they may block the eye area you need to analyze or treat.			
6. Use a magnifying light to examine the skin more thoroughly. A Wood's lamp or electronic imaging system may also be used.			
7. Look closely to determine the client's skin type, the conditions present, and the overall appearance.			
8. Touch the skin with the fingertips to feel its texture, its oil and water content, and its elasticity. Pay attention to the T-zone.			
9. Ask and listen. Ask questions about the skin's appearance, the client's health, and their lifestyle to gain a better understanding. Verbally describe to your client what you are finding in your analysis.			
10. Apply a toner and moisturizer or sunscreen to balance and protect the skin.			
11. Recommend a skin care plan that includes professional treatments and skin care products for a home care regimen. Giving the client a treatment plan in writing and including some skin care samples is a way to build your clientele.			
12. Record your findings and your recommendations in the client's chart—usually after the treatment is completed.			

CHAPTER 6
SKIN CARE PRODUCTS: CHEMISTRY, INGREDIENTS, AND SELECTION

EXPLAIN HOW SKIN CARE PRODUCTS AND INGREDIENTS ARE SIGNIFICANT TO ESTHETICIANS

SHORT ANSWER

1. Describe why an esthetician should study and have a thorough understanding of skin care products.

_____

_____

_____

_____

_____

_____

_____

_____

_____

_____

_____

DESCRIBE COSMETIC REGULATIONS, LAWS, AND PRODUCT SAFETY

FILL IN THE BLANK

2. It is critical for an esthetician to learn _____, _____, and _____ when it comes to cosmetic products.

FDA Regulations for Cosmetics

SHORT ANSWER

3. List the two most important laws pertaining to cosmetics marketed in the United States.

_____

_____

_____

_____

_____

_____

How does the law define a cosmetic?

SHORT ANSWER

4. What is a cosmetic according to the FD&C Act?

_____

_____

_____

_____

_____

_____

How does the law define a drug?

SHORT ANSWER

5. What is a drug according to the FD&C Act?

_____

_____

_____

_____

_____

_____

Can a product be both a cosmetic and a drug?

TRUE OR FALSE

6. For the following statements about cosmetics and drugs, circle T if true or F if false.

    T F   Some nonprescription medicated products have lower doses of active ingredients and meet the definitions of both cosmetics and drugs.

    T F   A cleanser is a cosmetic.

    T F   A moisturizer only meets the definition of a drug.

    T F   Makeup with sun protection is only a cosmetic.

What are cosmeceuticals?

MULTIPLE CHOICE

7. A cosmeceutical is _____.

    a. a legal term

    b. a lower-grade over-the-counter drug

    c. a skin care product or makeup that includes pharmaceutical-grade ingredients

    d. a cosmetic made by a pharmaceutical company

Product Labeling Laws and Regulations

TRUE OR FALSE

8. For the following statements about product labeling laws, circle T if true or F if false.

    T F   The label must list the company name, location, and ingredients.

    T F   Ingredients must be listed in ascending order.

    T F   Ingredients with a concentration of less than 1 percent must be listed alphabetically.

    T F   A fragrance must be listed as a fragrance.

INCI Names

FILL IN THE BLANK

9. The acronym INCI stands for _____.

10. INCI names are used _____.

Product Safety

SHORT ANSWER

11. When can the FDA take legal action against a cosmetic on the market?

_____

_____

_____

_____

_____

Adverse Reactions

SHORT ANSWER

12. List the general symptoms of an adverse reaction.

_____

_____

_____

_____

_____

13. Describe how to perform a patch test.

_____

_____

_____

_____

_____

14. What are the steps to follow if during a facial treatment the client's skin becomes excessively red?

_____

_____

_____

_____

_____

DISTINGUISH COSMETIC INGREDIENT SOURCES AND POPULAR TERMS

SHORT ANSWER

15. Where can cosmetic ingredients be derived from?

_____

_____

_____

_____

_____

Natural Versus Synthetic Ingredients

SHORT ANSWER

16. Describe the advantages of natural and synthetic ingredients.

_____

_____

_____

_____

Popular Terms

MATCHING

17. Match the description to the term.

a. natural	e. gluten-free	i. fragrance-free
b. organic	f. hypoallergenic	j. unscented
c. cruelty-free	g. noncomedogenic	
d. vegan	h. comedogenic	

_____ less likely to cause allergic reactions

_____ products not tested on animals

_____ should not contain animal ingredients

_____ does not clog pores

_____ grown without the use of pesticides or chemicals

_____ derived from natural sources

_____ related to celiac disease

_____ formulated to have no smell

_____ forms blackheads

_____ no ingredients added to provide a scent

DESCRIBE THE MAIN TYPES OF INGREDIENTS IN COSMETIC CHEMISTRY

SHORT ANSWER

18. Describe the two main categories of ingredients in cosmetic chemistry.

_____

_____

_____

_____

_____

Main Types of Ingredients in Product Formulations

MATCHING

19. Match the ingredient to its purpose.

a. water	i. traditional preservatives	q. aromatherapy
b. emollient	j. organic acid preservatives	r. color agents
c. surfactants	k. antioxidants	s. certified colors
d. delivery systems	l. chelating agents	t. lakes
e. vehicles	m. fragrances	u. noncertified colors
f. liposomes	n. synthetic fragrances	v. thickeners
g. polymers	o. natural fragrances	w. pH adjusters
h. preservatives	p. essential oils	f. solvents

_____ prevents bacteria, fungi, molds, and other microorganisms from living in a product

_____ reduce tension between the skin and the product

_____ bring key ingredients to a targeted depth of the skin and slowly release them

_____ helps keep other ingredients in a solution, helps to spread product across the skin, replenishes moisture

_____ used as advanced vehicles that release ingredients onto the skin's surface at a microscopically controlled rate

_____ helps place, spread, and keep substances on the skin and also lubricates skin's surface and guards the barrier function

_____ carries bases and spreading agents necessary for the formulation of a cosmetic

_____ used to distribute a product's key performance ingredients into the skin

_____ neutralizes the smell of a product

_____ fragrant "soul" of the plant, used for their natural aromas

_____ enhances product's visual appeal and changes the appearance of skin

_____ color additives synthesized mainly from raw materials obtained from petroleum; listed on labels as D&C or FD&C

_____ buffering agents that stabilize products

_____ color additives obtained primarily from mineral, plant, or animal sources

_____ insoluble pigments made by combining a dye with an inorganic material

_____ an ancient practice of using natural plant essences to promote health and well-being

_____ comprised of botanicals for use as scents in skin care product formulations

_____ extends the shelf life of a product and reduces the rate of oxidation in formulas when used as a preservative

_____ typically combined with natural alternatives for use as a preservative

_____ helps to suspend ingredients or to give products a specific consistency

_____ helps to dissolve ingredients

_____ boosts the efficacy of preservatives

_____ scents that can consist of as many as 200 ingredients; label will simply say "fragrance"

_____ used as a preservative that includes formaldehyde-releases and parabens

FILL IN THE BLANK

20. _____ ingredients originate from plants and can provide many benefits to support the health, texture, and integrity of the skin.

21. _____ can help skin appear brighter and can clear the path for other skin care products to work more effectively.

22. _____ are ingredients that physically polish away dead cells from the skin's surface.

23. _____ remove dead skin cells with the use of enzymes, hydroxy acids, and chemical compounds to aid in cell turnover.

24. _____ provide gentle exfoliation and dissolve keratin proteins within dead skin cells on the surface to make skin softer and smoother.

25. _____ are naturally occurring acids derived from fruit, nuts, milk, or sugars.

26. _____ is the beta hydroxy acid found in skin care products and is oil soluble so it can get into pores to cut through the oil that clogs them.

27. When applied to the skin, _____ , a vitamin A derivative, does not induce redness or irritation like products with high concentrations of hydroxy acids potentially can.

28. Botanicals are a very popular source of _____ , ingredients that provide and maintain a natural radiance and glow to the skin.

29. Lightening ingredients are also known as _____ suppressants, or tyrosinase inhibitors.

30. When applied topically, _____ , healing, and _____ ingredients provide vital nutrients and hydration to the skin and also play a crucial role in healing and repair.

31. _____, _____, and hydrophilic agents are ingredients that attract water to the skin's surface and lock water on the skin, reducing dehydration.

32. _____ are among the most effective ingredients for all skin types and conditions and when applied topically, they neutralize free radicals.

33. Deficiencies in your _____ intake can cause adverse effects on the skin, as they are essential to your health and body functions.

34. _____, like copper and zinc, provide therapeutic benefits when applied topically through skin care products.

35. In skin care products, many _____ ingredients are used to help reinforce the proteins naturally occurring in the skin and therefore revitalize the skin's building blocks so it becomes more resilient.

36. _____, a family of lipid molecules, replenish the natural lipids in skin that are lost from exposure to harsh environmental factors, from use of drying products, and during the natural aging process.

37. Botanicals such as calendula, chamomile, rose, and aloe vera have all been used in skin care for many years for their natural _____ properties.

38. Topically applied _____, considered one of the latest beauty breakthroughs, act to balance and retain healthy bacteria on your skin while combatting harmful bacteria.

39. _____ and beta glucans, normally derived from yeast cells, enhance the skin's defense mechanisms and stimulate cell metabolism.

40. _____, also called glycopolypeptides, are skin conditioning agents derived from carbohydrates and proteins.

41. _____, which promote skin tissue repair and regeneration, can be derived from human cells grown in a laboratory, as well as from nonhuman sources such as plants.

42. _____ help prevent ultraviolet radiation from harming the skin.

43. _____ sunscreen ingredients are organic compounds that work by absorbing UV rays into the skin, changing them to heat, then releasing them from the skin.

44. Physical sunscreen ingredients, also called mineral sunscreens, are inorganic mineral compounds that physically _____ or _____ ultraviolet radiation.

IDENTIFY BENEFICIAL INGREDIENTS FOR SKIN TYPES AND CONDITIONS

SHORT ANSWER

45. List the types of ingredients that can be used on all skin types and conditions.

_____

_____

_____

_____

_____

46. What is the goal in treating combination skin? List the types of ingredients used.

_____

_____

_____

_____

_____

47. What is the goal in treating dry skin? List the types of ingredients used.

_____

_____

_____

_____

_____

48. What is the goal in treating dehydrated skin? List the types of ingredients used.

_____

_____

_____

_____

_____

49. What is the goal in treating oily skin? List the types of ingredients used.

_____

_____

_____

_____

_____

50. What is the goal in treating acne/problematic skin? List the types of ingredients used.

_____

_____

_____

_____

_____

51. What is the goal in treating sensitive/reactive skin? List the types of ingredients used.

_____

_____

_____

_____

_____

52. What is the goal in treating hyperpigmentation? List the types of ingredients used.

_____

_____

_____

_____

_____

53. How do you treat mature/aging skin? List the types of ingredients used.

_____

_____

_____

_____

_____

SELECT APPROPRIATE PRODUCTS FOR FACIAL TREATMENTS AND HOME CARE USE

COLLAGE

Create a collage of products for facial treatments. Consider grouping them together based on their specific benefits. You may create your collage in the space below, use a separate sheet of paper, or assemble it digitally.

54. For each of the following products, find an example in a magazine or on the Internet, identify the type (if there is more than one), and list its benefits.

cleansers: _____

_____

_____

_____

_____

_____

toners: _____

_____

_____

_____

_____

exfoliants: _____

_____

_____

_____

_____

_____

masks: _____

_____

_____

_____

_____

_____

massage products: _____

_____

_____

_____

_____

_____

serums and ampoules: _____

_____

_____

_____

_____

moisturizers and hydrators: _____

_____

_____

_____

_____

specialty products for eyes and lips (one product for each): _____

_____

_____

_____

_____

sun protection: _____

_____

_____

_____

_____

RECOMMEND HOME CARE PRODUCTS WITH CONFIDENCE

SHORT ANSWER

55. Why is retailing important for an esthetician's job?

_____

_____

_____

_____

_____

Three Steps to Successful Retailing

SHORT ANSWER

56. List and describe the three steps to successful retailing

- _____
  _____
  _____
  _____
  _____

- _____
  _____
  _____
  _____
  _____

- _____
  _____
  _____
  _____

57. Research your favorite skin cleanser. Create a sales recommendation for that product and write it down using the three steps to successful retailing.

_____
_____
_____
_____
_____

SUMMARIZE THE POINTS TO CONSIDER WHEN CHOOSING A PROFESSIONAL SKIN CARE LINE

SHORT ANSWER

58. What do you need to consider when choosing a product line?

_____

_____

_____

_____

_____

_____

_____

_____

_____

_____

Product Prices and Costs

FILL IN THE BLANK

59. If you have a product priced at $50 for 2 ounces (56 g) and it is estimated to last six months, the cost per month is _____. The cost per week is _____. This is only _____ per day.

WORD REVIEW

WORD SEARCH

60. After determining the correct word from the clues provided, locate the words in the word search.

_____ helps heal damaged skin

_____ seaweed derivatives used as thickening agents

_____ derived from the root of the comfrey plant

_____ describes products that do not contain any water

_____ anti-inflammatory plant extract

_____ plant extract with calming and soothing properties

_____ liquids applied after cleansing to soothe and hydrate

_____ formed by a decomposition of oils or fats

_____ known as roll-off mask

_____ oil widely used in cosmetics

_____ skin-brightening agent

_____ insoluble pigments made by combining a dye with an inorganic material

_____ anti-irritant used for sensitive skin

_____ one of the fattiest and heaviest oils used as an emollient

_____ natural enzyme used for exfoliation and in enzyme peels

_____ natural form of vitamin A

_____ derived from olives

_____ reduces the activity of oil glands

_____ properties include enhancing the penetrative abilities of other substances

_____ extracted from the bark of the hamanelis shrub

C	A	C	A	I	B	E	R	R	Y	U	R	E	A	F
A	L	L	A	N	T	O	I	N	I	B	L	B	A	R
G	L	Y	C	E	R	I	N	A	T	A	O	S	A	E
A	A	G	H	A	A	U	A	T	A	J	R	L	E	S
N	P	A	A	T	O	R	S	A	O	A	U	A	A	H
H	R	P	M	E	A	E	A	J	A	D	A	K	L	E
Y	O	G	O	M	M	A	G	E	N	C	A	E	I	N
D	T	S	M	A	A	S	A	E	A	A	S	S	C	E
R	E	T	I	N	O	L	L	A	A	T	U	A	O	R
O	N	A	L	A	P	A	L	M	O	I	L	N	R	S
U	S	L	E	A	C	N	A	A	A	O	F	A	I	O
S	Q	U	A	L	A	N	E	R	O	N	U	A	C	N
T	C	P	A	P	A	Y	A	G	E	N	R	A	E	S
W	A	D	C	R	S	K	O	J	I	C	A	C	I	D
W	I	T	C	H	H	A	Z	E	L	I	L	A	A	A

DISCOVERIES AND ACCOMPLISHMENTS

In the space below, write notes about key concepts discussed in this chapter. Share your discoveries with some of the other students in your class and ask them if your notes are helpful. You may want to revise your discoveries based on good ideas shared by your peers.

Discoveries:

_____

_____

_____

_____

_____

_____

_____

_____

_____

_____

_____

_____

List at least three things you have accomplished since your last entry that relate to product ingredients, product chemistry, or selection.

Accomplishments:

_____

_____

_____

_____

_____

_____

_____

_____

_____

_____

EXAM REVIEW

MULTIPLE CHOICE

1. What are botanicals made from?

    a. plants and herbs

    b. chemicals

    c. animal fats

    d. recycled plastic

2. Which of the following is not a reason to have a thorough understanding of skin care products?

    a. to be able to explain why they're effective

    b. to explain how to properly use products at home

    c. to create your own products

    d. to set realistic expectations

3. What is a possible advantage of synthetic ingredients over natural ingredients?

    a. fewer allergic reactions

    b. shorter shelf life

    c. less environmental impact

    d. decreased chemical content

4. When is a manufacturer responsible for a client's allergic reaction to a product?

    a. when the product is purchased in bulk and repackaged by the salon

    b. when the product is used as an ingredient in a salon mixture

    c. when the product is taken directly from the manufacturer's packaging

    d. when the client ignores warnings on the product's label

5. When is the salon responsible for a client's allergic reaction to a product?

    a. when the client buys the product directly from the manufacturer

    b. when the product is purchased in bulk and repackaged by the salon

    c. when the client ignores warnings on the product's label

    d. when the product is taken directly from the manufacturer's packaging

6. What is not an area requiring approval from the Food and Drug Administration (FDA)?

    a. cosmetics manufacturing

    b. cosmetics safety

    c. cosmetics labelling

    d. cosmetics claims

7. What term refers to skin-freshening lotions with a low alcohol content?

    a. moisturizers

    b. antibiotics

    c. fresheners

    d. conditioners

8. What is not among the purposes of functional ingredients in cosmetic products?

    a. allowing products to spread

    b. giving products body and texture

    c. making products affordable

    d. giving products specific form

9. Which ingredients can be used to treat dehydrated skin?

    a. humectants

    b. exfoliants

    c. hydroxy acids

    d. brighteners

10. What term refers to an exfoliating cream that is rubbed off the skin?

    a. humectant

    b. emulsifier

    c. gommage

    d. paraben

11. What are hydrators?

    a. machines used to apply water to the skin's surface

    b. machines used to extract water from the skin's surface

    c. ingredients that attract water to the skin's surface

    d. ingredients that repel water from the skin's surface

12. What are alpha hydroxy acids?

    a. products that exfoliate by loosening bonds between dead cells

    b. products that exfoliate by tightening bonds between living cells

    c. the active ingredients in most acne-treatment medications

    d. the active ingredients in most dandruff-control shampoos

13. What type of product does not sometimes include alcohol?

    a. perfume

    b. lotion

    c. astringent

    d. paraffin mask

14. What is an ampoule?

    a. small, sealed vial

    b. needle used for injections

    c. popular botanical cream

    d. family of chemical products

15. What is aromatherapy?

    a. practice of focusing massage on the nose and nostrils

    b. therapeutic use of plant aromas and essential oils

    c. therapeutic use of scented candles in the treatment room

    d. practice of focusing acupuncture on the nose and nostrils

16. What are astringents?

    a. cotton pads used to dab excess sebum from the surface of the skin

    b. cotton pads used to dab excess lymph from the surface of the skin

    c. oil-laden liquids used to increase the oiliness of the skin

    d. liquids that help remove excess oil on the skin

17. What are ingredients derived from plants called?

    a. chemicals

    b. pharmaceuticals

    c. pentacostals

    d. botanicals

18. What are ceramides?

    a. astringents that have moisturizing and antibacterial properties

    b. family of lipid materials

    c. bacteria that cause itching in the surface of the skin

    d. clusters of dead skin cells that clog follicles and cause comedones

19. What plant extract has calming and soothing properties?

   a. blackcurrant

   b. chamomile

   c. ginseng

   d. honeybush

20. What are lakes?

   a. insoluble pigments

   b. botanical moisturizers

   c. botanical emulsifiers

   d. insoluble antioxidants

21. What is not true of polymers?

   a. They are chemical compounds.

   b. They are botanicals.

   c. They are formed by small molecules.

   d. They release substances at a microscopically controlled rate.

22. What function do preservatives perform?

   a. give products the desired color, shape, and form

   b. give products the desired efficacy and strength

   c. activate products once they are applied to the skin

   d. inhibit the growth of microorganism

23. What is the vitamin of which retinol is the natural form?

   a. vitamin A

   b. vitamin B

   c. vitamin C

   d. vitamin D

24. What vitamin has not been used in skin care products as an antioxidant?

   a. vitamin A

   b. vitamin B

   c. vitamin C

   d. vitamin E

25. What are liposomes?
    a. open-lipid bilayer spheres
    b. open-lipid unilayer spores
    c. closed-lipid bilayer spheres
    d. closed-lipid unilayer spores

26. What is mechanical exfoliation?
    a. physical method of rubbing dead cells off the skin
    b. use of machines to push product deeper into the skin
    c. physical method of drawing pus from a whitehead
    d. use of machines to draw pus from a whitehead

27. What is papaya used for?
    a. exfoliation
    b. moisturizing
    c. hydration
    d. pigmentation

28. Which of the following is not a step to successful retailing?
    a. provide product education
    b. present precise instructions
    c. practice professional follow-up
    d. prepare a business plans with high mark-ups

29. What are peptides?
    a. chains of red blood cells
    b. chains of white blood cells
    c. chains of fibroblasts
    d. chains of amino acids

30. What are performance ingredients?
    a. ingredients included to elongate the shelf life of products
    b. ingredients used to give products distinct shape and texture
    c. ingredients that cause actual changes in the appearance of the skin
    d. ingredients that stimulate blood circulation and increase energy

31. What is a chelating agent?
    a. chemical added to improve the thickness of a product
    b. chemical added to improve the efficacy of the preservative
    c. chemical added to soften the aroma of a product
    d. chemical added to increase the grit of a product

32. What do clay masks do as they dry and tighten?
    a. seal follicles
    b. rupture comedones
    c. extract facial hairs
    d. draw impurities to the surface

33. What is coenzyme Q10?
    a. antioxidant
    b. exfoliant
    c. preservative
    d. emulsifier

34. What is the term for substances such as mineral dyes that give products color?
    a. color additives
    b. color ingredients
    c. color agents
    d. chromophores

35. What term refers to products intended to improve the skin's health and appearance?
    a. cosmetics
    b. cosmeceuticals
    c. epidermals
    d. estheticals

36. What are detergents a type of?
    a. surfactant
    b. emollient
    c. antioxidant
    d. exfoliant

37. What do emulsifiers cause to mix in order to form an emulsion?

    a. oil and lymph

    b. oil and water

    c. lymph and water

    d. lymph and sebum

38. What is a good way to determine actual product costs?

    a. break down the product costs by number of bottles in the box

    b. break down the purchase price into daily and weekly costs

    c. break down the product costs by the number of clients who use the product

    d. break down the purchase price into costs per ounce

39. What are fatty acids?

    a. excessive sebum discharges common in overweight clients

    b. excessive lymph discharges common in overweight clients

    c. antioxidant ingredients derived solely from animal fats

    d. lubricant ingredients derived from plant oils or animal fats

40. What function do fragrances perform?

    a. giving products their color

    b. giving products their scent

    c. giving products their taste

    d. giving products their texture

41. Which term is often used loosely because there is no specific legal definition?

    a. organic

    b. natural

    c. vegan

    d. cruelty-free

42. What describes natural-sourced ingredients that are grown without the use of pesticides or chemicals?

    a. organic

    b. natural

    c. vegan

    d. cruelty-free

43. This product is not tested on animals at any stage of the production process.

    a. organic

    b. natural

    c. vegan

    d. cruelty-free

44. This product does not contain any animal ingredients or animal by-products.

    a. cruelty-free

    b. hypoallergenic

    c. vegan

    d. gluten-free

45. To receive a gluten-free label, a product must have less than _____ parts per million of gluten.

    a. 20

    b. 40

    c. 60

    d. 80

46. Which products are less likely to cause allergic reactions?

    a. comedogenic

    b. hypoallergenic

    c. noncomedogenic

    d. unscented

47. Which of the following statements is true about fragrance-free products?

    a. They have no smell.

    b. More ingredients have been added to mask the smell.

    c. The smell has been neutralized.

    d. No additional ingredients have been added to provide a fragrance.

48. Which of the following ingredients would not be used to treat combination skin?

    a. emollients

    b. humectants

    c. exfoliants

    d. oil balancing

49.   What is the goal in treating dehydrated skin?

    a.   to promote a healthy oil–water balance

    b.   to provide skin restoring ingredients

    c.   to retain inner moisture by preventing TEWL

    d.   to keep pores from becoming clogged

50.   When treating sensitive skin, you want to find products with what type of ingredients?

    a.   calming

    b.   brightening

    c.   restoring

    d.   rejuvenating

51.   If you are trying to prevent further darkening of pigmented areas, then you are most likely treating which skin condition?

    a.   mature/aging

    b.   hyperpigmented

    c.   combination

    d.   acne/problematic

52.   What is the most important part of any treatment or home care regimen?

    a.   tailored toward client preferences

    b.   effective for a person's individual needs

    c.   reasonable in price

    d.   easy to find and purchase

53.   What determines the quality and effectiveness of professional products?

    a.   the method and length of application

    b.   manufacturing process, not the ingredients

    c.   ingredients alone, not the manufacturing process

    d.   ingredients' source and the manufacturing process

54.   Which of the following is not a consideration when choosing a product line?

    a.   Is the range of products versatile?

    b.   What support in training and education does the manufacturer provide?

    c.   How many colors does it come in?

    d.   Is the packaging appealing and easy to use?

55.   What is the general percentage markup for retail products in a salon?

    a.   50 percent

    b.   25 percent

    c.   75 percent

    d.   100 percent

CHAPTER 7
THE TREATMENT ROOM

EXPLAIN WHY TREATMENT ROOM PREPARATION IS AN INTEGRAL PART OF PROVIDING TREATMENTS

SHORT ANSWER

1. Explain four reasons an esthetician should have a thorough understanding of the treatment room.

_____

_____

_____

_____

_____

_____

_____

_____

_____

_____

REVIEW THE ELEMENTS OF AN ESTHETICIAN'S PROFESSIONAL APPEARANCE

SHORT ANSWER

2. Kendra is about to have her first day at work as an esthetician. Describe how she might portray a professional appearance.

_____

_____

_____

_____

_____

Professional Image Checklist

SHORT ANSWER

3. List and describe seven elements of an esthetician's professional image.

_____

_____

_____

_____

_____

OUTLINE ESSENTIAL ROOM AND STATION STRUCTURAL FEATURES

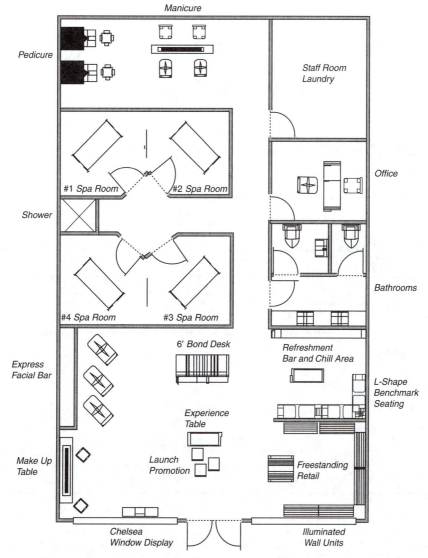

Structural Features

MATCHING

4. Match the essential structural features in an esthetics room to its description.

a. size	d. running water
b. proper ventilation	e. washable flooring and workstation surfaces
c. electrical outlets	f. proper lighting

_____ Treatment rooms should have a minimum of four of these.

_____ This must be functioning and calibrated for two or more people.

_____ This should be made of nonabsorbent washable synthetic materials.

_____ This should be large enough to ensure proper movement.

_____ This should be able to be increased or decreased during skin analysis and product removal.

_____ This is essential for thorough removal of facial and body products.

DESCRIBE THE IDEAL AMBIENCE, FURNITURE, AND EQUIPMENT FOR FACIALS

SHORT ANSWER

5. Stacey is opening a spa. Describe what she may want her clients' first impression to be when they walk in the door.

_____

_____

_____

_____

_____

Ambience

SHORT ANSWER

6. Describe how features in Stacey's spa could engage all five of the senses.

_____

_____

_____

_____

_____

A Checklist of Furniture and Equipment

COLLAGE

7. Design your own treatment room, using photos from magazines, websites, or your personal collection to show the supplies and furniture that you have selected for the treatment room. Design on a separate poster board or piece of paper, or make a digital collage.

Ergonomics in the Treatment Room

SHORT ANSWER

8. Find a picture of a stool or describe in the space below one that you would like to have in your treatment room. Then describe how it is ergonomically correct.

_____

_____

_____

_____

_____

9. List two ways to arrange the equipment in the treatment room for proper ergonomics.

_____

_____

_____

_____

Costs of Starting Your Own Business

SHORT ANSWER

10. You are looking at a potential location to open your first spa. The rent is $21 per square foot (annually), and the space is 1,800 square feet. How much rent would you pay each year? Each month?

_____

_____

_____

_____

_____

11. Equipment for your salon will cost anywhere from $7,000 to $10,000. How much money will you spend over the course of the first year with rent and equipment?

_____

_____

_____

_____

PROPERLY MANAGE TREATMENT ROOM SUPPLIES AND PRODUCTS

SHORT ANSWER

12. Describe how you would control inventory in your dispensary.

_____

_____

_____

_____

Facial Treatment Supplies and Implements

LABELING

13. List the facial treatment supplies for basic facial products that you will need in the order of use on the lines provided below. On the following page, draw those supplies on the provided cart.

A) _____   I) _____

B) _____   J) _____

C) _____   K) _____

D) _____   L) _____

E) _____   M) _____

F) _____   N) _____

G) _____   O) _____

H) _____   P) _____

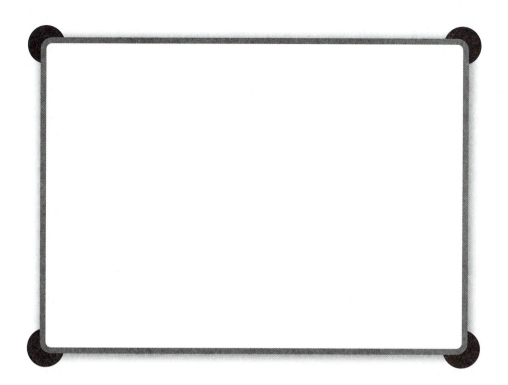

Single-Use Items

SHORT ANSWER

14. Describe how a single-use item is different from a multi-use item.

_____

_____

_____

_____

_____

15. Give five examples of single-use items.

1. _____

2. _____

3. _____

4. _____

5. _____

16. Give five examples of multi-use items.

1. _____

2. _____

3. _____

4. _____

5. _____

Products

SHORT ANSWER

17. Sara is setting up her cart for a facial appointment. List 10 basic products that she will put on her cart.

_____

_____

_____

_____

_____

_____

_____

_____

_____

_____

_____

_____

_____

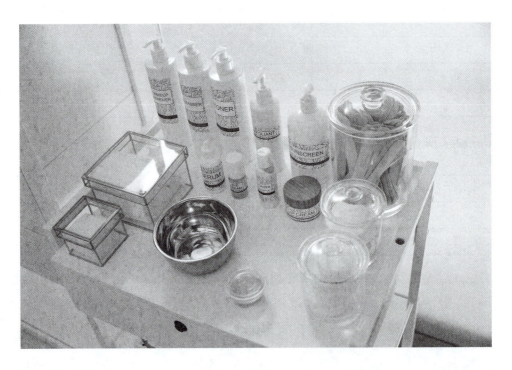

BE ABLE TO SET UP A FACIAL TREATMENT AREA—FACIAL BAR OR STATION

SHORT ANSWER

18. How is a facial bar or station different from a treatment room?

_____

_____

_____

_____

_____

_____

_____

_____

_____

_____

PREPARE THE TREATMENT ROOM FOR SERVICES

SHORT ANSWER

19. You've just arrived at work. Create a setup checklist for the treatment room that you can refer to and that will help you memorize the steps. The first step is provided to get you started. The number of steps you fill out depends on your personal checklist.

   1. Look at your schedule for the day to see what supplies are needed.

   2. _____

   3. _____

   4. _____

   5. _____

   6. _____

   7. _____

   8. _____

   9. _____

   10. _____

11. _____

12. _____

13. _____

14. _____

15. _____

Setting Out Single-Use Items

SHORT ANSWER

20. Describe four steps for setting out single-use items.

_____

_____

_____

_____

_____

_____

_____

_____

Setting Up the Dressing Area

SHORT ANSWER

21. How would you set up your client's dressing area?

_____

_____

_____

_____

_____

_____

Procedure 7–1: Pre-Service—Preparing the Treatment Room

LABELING

22. Describe what is happening in each of the following pictures.

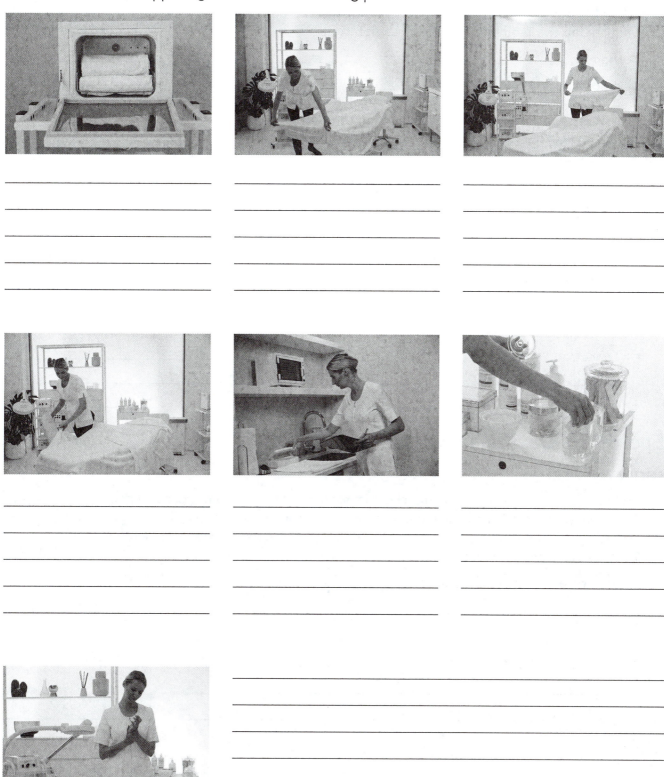

PROPERLY CLEAN AND DISINFECT THE TREATMENT ROOM

SHORT ANSWER

23. What are the two methods of proper infection control?

   Method 1: _____

   Method 2: _____

Appropriate Handling of Single-Use Items

SHORT ANSWER

24. Describe the appropriate handling of single-use items.

   - **Gloves:** _____
     _____
     _____

   - **Clean supplies:** _____
     _____
     _____

   - **Lancets:** _____
     _____
     _____

End-of-the-Day Clean-Up

SHORT ANSWER

25. Create your end-of-the-day clean-up checklist for the treatment room for your school. Repetitive practice will help you memorize the steps. The first step is provided to get you started. The number of steps you fill out depends on your personal checklist. (Note that all 10 steps may not be needed.)

   1. Turn off and unplug all equipment.

   2. _____

   3. _____

   4. _____

   5. _____

   6. _____

   7. _____

   8. _____

   9. _____

   10. _____

Procedure 7–2: Post-Service—Clean-Up and Preparation for the Next Client

SHORT ANSWER

26. Describe the difference between the end-of-service checklist and the end-of-the-day checklist.

_____

_____

_____

_____

_____

WORD REVIEW

MATCHING

27. Match each term to its definition.

a. dispensary	c. implements
b. facial station	d. trolley

_____ tools used by technicians to perform services

_____ skin care treatment area within the reception or retail area of the facility

_____ a rolling cart that holds tools, supplies, and products

_____ room or area used for mixing products and storing supplies

DISCOVERIES AND ACCOMPLISHMENTS

Compare the checklists you have made with those made by your classmates, and write down any differences in the space below. Discuss any differences between your lists, and work together to make sure that each person has a comprehensive list.

Discoveries:

_____

_____

_____

_____

_____

_____

_____

_____

_____

_____

_____

_____

List at least three things you have accomplished since your last entry that relate to your career goals.

Accomplishments:

_____

_____

_____

_____

_____

_____

_____

_____

_____

_____

_____

_____

_____

EXAM REVIEW

MULTIPLE CHOICE

1. What should you wash your hands with before touching clean supplies?

    a. soap and warm water

    b. chemical disinfectant

    c. autoclave steam

    d. harsh exfoliant

2. What should you do with single-use items as you prepare for a treatment?

    a. place them on a countertop in descending size order

    b. set them on a clean towel in the order they will be used

    c. place them on a countertop in ascending size order

    d. set them on a clean towel with containers open and ready

3. Sandra has an appointment with a new client, and she is not sure if the client has ever had a facial or waxing before. What should she do to make sure the client knows what to do?

    a. remain silent while the client figures out for themselves how to do things

    b. ask the receptionist to educate the client before treatments

    c. prepare a brochure explaining what to expect

    d. explain to the client where to put belongings and how to put on the wrap

4. Why should you wear gloves for all infection control procedures?

    a. to prevent contamination

    b. to protect your skin from strong chemicals

    c. to prevent contamination and protect your skin from strong chemicals

    d. it is not necessary to wear gloves for all infection control procedures

5. What do paper towels, tissues, and vinyl gloves have in common?

    a. They are multi-use items.

    b. They are single-use items.

    c. They are disinfecting products.

    d. They are massage products.

6. What piece of equipment is also known as an operator's stool?

    a. receptionist's chair

    b. esthetician's chair

    c. manager's chair

    d. client's chair

7. What is a sharps container?

    a. disinfectant-filled jar in which fresh hair shears are stored

    b. plastic case in which unused injectables are stored

    c. biohazard container for disposable needles and sharp objects

    d. special wastebasket for breakable items such as glass

8. What is a dispensary?

    a. drawer at the reception desk for storing retail products

    b. printing machine at your station that produces service tickets

    c. room or area used for mixing products and storing supplies

    d. another name for the pharmacy closest to your salon

9. What are implements?

    a. multi-use or single-use tools

    b. ingrown hairs

    c. contraindications

    d. garments worn by clients

10. What is the result of planning and preparing a well-stocked and organized treatment room?

    a. completing treatments as quickly as possible

    b. providing a service

    c. providing perfect treatment results

    d. functioning efficiently and providing good service

11. Why is it important for estheticians/students to maintain clean treatment rooms?

    a. showcasing new products

    b. maintaining inventory

    c. ensuring client safety and compliance with laws

    d. cleaning treatment rooms is not the job of estheticians

12. What is a benefit of being prepared?

    a. You never encounter surprises.

    b. You never have problems at work.

    c. You project a calm, confident image.

    d. You do everything well.

13. When in the process of performing services do you plan and prepare the treatment room?

    a. at the beginning

    b. at the end

    c. once the client arrives

    d. once the treatment is underway

14. What is the function of a magnifying lamp or light?

    a. directing LED beams

    b. analyzing the skin

    c. heating up product for deeper penetration into the dermis

    d. blocking LED beams

15. Linnea knows that during the holidays, she usually sees an uptick in demand for services. What should she do to keep her spa ready for walk-ins or unexpected requests?

    a. keep massage oil on her hands

    b. keep water running all day

    c. keep wax heaters on all day

    d. avoid taking breaks or lunches

16. What is **NOT** a spa area in which supplies are regularly kept?

    a. work station

    b. treatment room

    c. reception desk

    d. dispensary

17. What should you use to disperse products from jars?

    a. fingers

    b. scissors

    c. tongs

    d. spatulas

18. What should you have among your facial supplies in order to provide neck support for the client?

    a. sponge

    b. pillow or rolled hand towel

    c. medical neck brace

    d. bed warmer

19. How long, approximately, is required for pre-heating of towel warmers and steamers?

    a. 5 minutes

    b. 15 minutes

    c. 30 minutes

    d. 60 minutes

20. When should you check the water level on the steamer?

    a. before preheating and regularly thereafter

    b. only before preheating

    c. only when it goes past the fill line

    d. checking the water level is unnecessary

21. What is true of waste containers?

    a. They should never be used in the treatment room.

    b. They require a self-closing lid and foot pedal.

    c. They require the same clean-up as a sink or basin.

    d. They should be used to dispose of all implements as part of the service.

22. Why should you place a blanket over the clean linens that you place on the treatment table?

    a. to keep the sheets protected from stains

    b. to keep the client warm and comfortable

    c. only to keep the client comfortable

    d. to cut down on how often linens must be cleaned

23. What is true about estheticians and well-groomed hair?

    a. It must be kept short.

    b. If worn long, it does not need to be pulled back.

    c. It is okay if it touches the clients on occasion.

    d. Healthy hair is linked to healthy skin.

24. When working in a salon or spa, is it acceptable to wear nail polish?

    a. Yes, especially if it is bold, bright polish.

    b. Yes, if it is light in color and permitted by your employer.

    c. Yes, as it is marketing tool for the latest colors and designs.

    d. Yes, so you can demonstrate how long the polish lasts even when you are in chemicals all day.

25. How can you convey a positive attitude?

   a. a timid smile

   b. limited eye contact

   c. a quick handshake

   d. good posture

26. Which structural feature is described in square feet?

   a. area

   b. proper ventilation

   c. flooring

   d. lighting

27. Which structural feature must follow guidelines provided by the Occupational Safety and Health Administration (OSHA)?

   a. size

   b. ventilation

   c. flooring

   d. lighting

28. Treatment rooms should have a minimum of _____ electrical outlet(s).

   a. three

   b. four

   c. two

   d. one

29. What can you do if you do not have running water in the treatment room?

   a. bring in two bowls of water and a hot towel cabinet

   b. offer only services that do not require water

   c. have the client step outside the room to rinse off products

   d. look for alternative locations that will allow you to have water in the treatment room

30. How many of the senses should a proper spa experience engage?

   a. two

   b. three

   c. four

   d. five

31.   What piece of equipment sterilizes other equipment?

   a.   steamer

   b.   galvanic machine

   c.   autoclave

   d.   hot cabi

32.   In a short break between clients it is a good idea to _____.

   a.   stretch and take 12 deep breaths

   b.   return all missed personal calls

   c.   enjoy a quick snack

   d.   check your email

33.   What is a bolster used for?

   a.   disinfecting

   b.   dispersing products

   c.   extractions

   d.   back support

34.   Which of the following treatments cannot be done at a facial station?

   a.   eye treatment

   b.   intensive peel

   c.   sheet mask

   d.   beard treatment

35.   Which of the following is true about facial stations?

   a.   They are usually located in the rear of the salon.

   b.   Full-body massages can be performed at these stations.

   c.   The client does not need to disrobe for these treatments.

   d.   Men's treatments are not done in these areas.

36.   When scheduling her clients, Toby always takes into account time to prepare the treatment room. How long should she *ideally* allow to set up for a service?

   a.   5 minutes

   b.   10 minutes

   c.   15 minutes

   d.   30 minutes

37. How long does it typically take to clean up after a service?

     a. 5 to 10 minutes

     b. 10 to 15 minutes

     c. 15 to 30 minutes

     d. 30 to 45 minutes

38. What is the correct order of products for an application procedure?

     a. cleanser, massage cream or lotion, mask, toner, moisturizer, and other products

     b. cleanser, moisturizer, massage cream or lotion, mask, toner, and other products

     c. cleanser, toner, massage cream or lotion, mask, moisturizer, and other products

     d. cleanser, mask, massage cream or lotion, toner, moisturizer, and other products

39. When setting up the dressing area, what is one thing you should never do?

     a. get water or tea ready, as it might not be at the client's preferred beverage

     b. assume the client will want a robe and slippers

     c. explain what clothes need to be removed and how to put the gown on

     d. touch a client's jewelry or assist them with removal of the jewelry

40. To avoid cross-contamination, how do you roll used linens?

     a. Roll them outward, so you can see which linens are dirty.

     b. It does not matter, since they will be placed in the laundry hamper.

     c. Roll them inward, so the dirty side is inside the laundry bundle.

     d. First shake them onto the floor, then roll them inward.

PROCEDURE 7–1: PRE-SERVICE: PREPARING THE TREATMENT ROOM

Evaluate your practical skills.

CRITERIA	COMPETENT	NEEDS WORK	IMPROVEMENT PLAN
A. Review the Daily Schedule			
1. Review your client schedule for the day and decide which products you are likely to need for each service. Make sure you have enough of all the products you will be using that day. You may have to retrieve additional product from the dispensary. This is also a good time to refresh your mind about each repeat client you will be seeing that day and their individual concerns.			
2. Retrieve the client's intake form or service record card and review it. If the appointment is for a new client, the client will need a new intake form.			
B. Equipment Preparation			
3. Turn on the wax heater as needed. Check and adjust the temperature.			
4. Preheat the towel warmer and put in wet towels. Note: Towels should not be dripping wet.			
5. Preheat the steamer. First check the steamer water level (it should be just slightly below the fill line). If necessary, refill the steamer. Follow the manufacturer's directions for care.			
6. Preheat any other equipment needed.			
C. Prepare the Treatment Table			
7. Wash your hands with soap and warm water before setting up and touching clean items.			
8. Place one sheet lengthwise on the treatment table.			
9. Place one hand towel lengthwise on top of the sheet at the head of the bed. Lay out another hand towel for placement over the décolleté on the upper chest area if applicable.			
10. Place the second sheet lengthwise on top of the first.			
11. Fold the top one-quarter of the second sheet back horizontally. Then fold the sheet diagonally across the bed.			
12. Place a blanket on top of the linens to keep the client warm and comfortable.			
13. Have a clean headband and gown or wrap ready for the client.			
14. Have a bolster and pillow available.			

D. Setting Up Supplies			
15. Check to make sure the disinfectant is ready. Wet disinfectants are filled and changed according to the manufacturer's instructions (check to see that the strength is maintained by regular refilling).			
16. Place supplies on a clean towel (paper or cloth) on the clean and disinfected workstation. Put out supplies in the order used, line up neatly, and if any supplies or products are uncovered, cover with another towel until you are ready to use them.			
17. Set up the professional trolley with supplies and disposables. See the list of materials needed and the visual for reference.			
E. Setting Up the Dressing Area			
18. Dispense only the amount of product needed for the service.			
19. Arrange a clean robe or spa wrap folded on a small table for the client to change into. (Note: for a facial bar, clothing is not removed.)			
20. Have cold water or tea water ready for the client.			
F. Preparing for the Client			
21. Organize yourself by taking care of your personal needs before the client arrives—stretch, use the restroom, get a drink of water, return personal calls—so you can focus your full attention on their needs. Remember to turn off electronic devices to eliminate any distractions. Take a moment to clear your head of all your personal concerns and issues.			
22. Referencing Procedure 5–3: Proper Hand Washing located in Milady Standard Foundations, wash your hands before going to greet your client.			
23. Your client has arrived! Proceed to follow the steps outlined in Procedure 8–1: Pre-Service: Prepare the Client for Treatment.			

PROCEDURE 7–2: POST-SERVICE: CLEAN-UP AND PREPARATION FOR THE NEXT CLIENT

Evaluate your practical skills.

CRITERIA	COMPETENT	NEEDS WORK	IMPROVEMENT PLAN
A. End-of-Service Checklist			
1. Create an end of service checklist that works for your space. Not everyone will complete the post-service steps in the same order.			
2. Place all soiled laundry linens (towels and sheets) in a covered receptacle.			
3. Discard any used disposables into a covered trash container.			
4. Disposable extraction lancets go in a sharps disposal container. (Check OSHA and state rules for proper handling.)			
5. Wipe down all equipment with an EPA-approved disinfectant.			
6. Clean trolley and workstation surfaces. Clean and disinfect the bottom tray and the inside of the towel warmer after removing all used items.			
7. Reset products and disposable items and replenish clean robes and spa wraps.			
8. Use an antibacterial dish soap and warm water to wash the used bowl(s). Rinse and dry thoroughly.			
9. Change linen on the treatment table.			
B. End-of-Day Checklist			
1. Complete the end of service checklist and check the schedule for the next shift or workday.			
2. Use an end-of-day checklist to make sure you do not forget anything.			
3. Turn off and unplug all equipment.			
4. Leave the towel-warmer door open to dry and empty the tray underneath before cleaning and disinfecting it.			
5. Clean anything that has not been cleaned after the last service, including the equipment, bed, sink, counters, and doorknobs.			
6. Refill all containers, supplies, and the steamer.			
7. Check floors; sweep or mop as required. Check for wax spills.			
8. Empty waste containers. Replace with clean trash liners.			
9. Remove personal items from the area.			

CHAPTER 8
FACIAL TREATMENTS

EXPLAIN THE IMPORTANCE OF FACIAL TREATMENTS

SHORT ANSWER

1. Sumi has seen an increase in requests for facial appointments at her salon. Knowing that this a growing trend, she wants to continue to offer services her clients find helpful. What are two things she can do to meet the needs of her clients, so her clients understand why facials are a necessity, not just nice to have?

_____

_____

_____

_____

_____

_____

_____

_____

_____

_____

DESCRIBE THE BENEFITS OF A FACIAL TREATMENT

SHORT ANSWER

2. Shannon's friend, Alexi, is coming into the spa to get her first facial. How can Shannon describe the experience and benefits of a facial to inform her friend?

_____

_____

_____

_____

_____

_____

_____

_____

LIST THE ESSENTIAL SKILLS NEEDED TO SUCCESSFULLY PERFORM FACIALS

MIND MAPPING

3. Write all of the things that you can do to be successful at providing facials that meet client expectations or that *exceed* those expectations.

_____

_____

_____

_____

_____

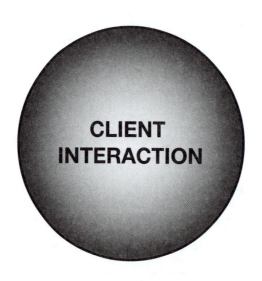

CLIENT INTERACTION

PERFORM THE FACIAL SETUP PROCEDURES

SHORT ANSWER

4. Write steps describing how to greet a new client, including brief instructions for changing and assisting the client onto the facial bed. Space has been provided for you.

1. _____
   _____
   _____

2. _____
   _____
   _____

3. _____
   _____
   _____

4. _____
   _____
   _____

5. _____
   _____
   _____

6. _____
   _____
   _____

7. _____
   _____
   _____

8. _____
   _____
   _____

9. _____
   _____
   _____

EXPLAIN THE KEY STEPS OF THE BASIC FACIAL TREATMENT

FILL IN THE BLANK

5. It is Nina's first day at her new job. Claudia, her new manager, has taken the time to share the salon's procedures with Nina. Pretend you are Claudia and fill in the missing steps for Nina. Some have been provided for you.

   1. Client consultation, including review of contraindications

   2. _____

   3. Initial skin analysis and continues client consultation; treatment plan creation

   4. _____

   5. In-depth skin analysis

   6. Exfoliation procedure

   7. _____

   8. Softening with steam or warm towels

   9. _____

   10. _____

   11. Toner

   12. Serums, eye treatments, and lip treatments

   13. Moisturizer

   14. _____

   15. Service completion, including post-consultation and home care

The Initial Consultation and Analysis

ROLE PLAY

6. Choose another student as your partner and conduct a facial treatment consultation on each other. Record your results in the sample intake form provided on page 184. This is a way to get familiar with the type of information you will learn about your clients.

7. Apply your knowledge from activity 6 to point out any contraindications for services. Then create a treatment plan to treat the concerns they may have. Fill out your choices for products you would use in the service in the chart provided on the following page.

Treatment Plan

Steps	Procedures
Cleansing	☐ Cream ☐ Liquid ☐ Mousse ☐ Gel ☐ Steam hot or cold
Exfoliation	☐ AHA ☐ BHA ☐ Enzymes ☐ Microdermabrasion ☐ Rotary brush
Advanced Protocols	☐ Galvanic ☐ High frequency ☐ Microcurrent
Massage	☐ Oil ☐ Cream ☐ Gel ☐ Serum
Mask(s)	☐ Sheet ☐ Cream ☐ Mud/Clay ☐ Alginate ☐ Mineral

Exfoliation Product or Mask

FILL IN THE BLANK

8. Write in the type of exfoliation based on the clues provided: mechanical, manual, or chemical exfoliation.

_____ a. removes dead skin by manipulation with the fingertips

_____ b. microdermabrasion

_____ c. enzyme

_____ d. use of honey and jojoba beads with fingers

_____ e. alpha hydroxy acids

_____ f. rotary brush

_____ g. rice bran to polish away dead cells

_____ h. salicylic acid

Completing the Service

FILL IN THE BLANK

9. Fill in the missing steps when it comes to completing a facial service:

1. Explain to the client what to do next (for example, get dressed).

2. _____

3. Show the client which products you recommend.

4. Ask them what products they would like to take home with them.

5. _____

6. Explain that you will record the products you recommend in their file.

7. Schedule the next appointment and recommend other services you believe would benefit them.

8. _____

9. Be sure to record service information, observations, and product recommendations on the client record and file.

DESCRIBE HOW TO CONSULT CLIENTS ON HOME CARE

SHORT ANSWER

10. Jasmine's manager, Olivia, noticed that many of Jasmine's facial clients have been purchasing skin care products. Olivia has asked Jasmine to describe how she presents home care to clients. Write four methods that Jasmine likely uses to effectively advise her clients on skin care.

- _____
  _____
  _____

- _____
  _____
  _____

- _____
  _____
  _____

- _____
  _____
  _____

The Art of Recommendation

ROLE PLAY

11. Partner with a class member. Pretend you have the opportunity to recommend products to your client after a service. Practice with your classmate what you would say and how you would start the conversation. In your role-playing, apply your knowledge of making recommendations and what you know of your client as discussed in the chapter. Afterward list your strengths and room for improvement and discuss ways to improve the conversation.

STRENGTHS

_____
_____
_____
_____

ROOM FOR IMPROVEMENT

_____

_____

_____

_____

_____

DISCUSS VARIATIONS OF THE BASIC FACIAL

FILL IN THE BLANK

12. Place the following steps of a basic facial in the correct order, from 1 to start. Two of the steps are not necessary. Leave these out.

_____ Properly drape the client and wash your hands.

_____ Apply a mask for approximately 10 minutes.

_____ Book the client's next visit.

_____ Massage.

_____ Perform a full facial cleansing.

_____ Analyze the skin with a magnifying lamp.

_____ Apply serums, eye and lip treatments.

_____ Place protective ointment around the eyes, corners of the nose, and the lips.

_____ Perform exfoliation. Remove exfoliant and tone skin.

_____ Perform extractions.

_____ Remove the mask.

_____ Recommend initial home care products and complete the home care chart.

_____ Apply a moisturizer and sunscreen for daytime.

_____ Perform a cleansing to remove makeup.

_____ Apply toner.

_____ Steam the face.

_____ Apply protective eyewear for yourself.

OUTLINE THE TREATMENT GOALS FOR SKIN TYPES/CONDITIONS

FILL IN THE BLANK

13. Fill in the blanks with the appropriate words. Some sentences may have more than one answer.

Dry Skin

FILL IN THE BLANK

a. Dry skin can appear _____, _____, and dull in color.

b. Treatment goals are similar for dry and _____ skin.

c. When treating dry skin, use a _____ or _____ to exfoliate the face.

d. When treating dry skin with a mask, use _____, or _____ and natural ingredients masks can be used.

Dehydrated Skin

FILL IN THE BLANK

e. Moisturizing creams with a(n) _____ base are recommended for dry skin types.

f. Skin may have a sufficient amount of oil but still feel dry and flaky due to _____.

g. Dehydrated skin may appear _____ but is _____ to the touch.

Mature or Aging Skin

FILL IN THE BLANK

h. Extreme weight loss can result in loss of _____ and _____ skin.

i. Mature clients' skin can be improved, but the natural aging process cannot be _____.

j. Treatment goals for mature skin are to _____ and _____.

k. When treating mature skin, a(n) _____ mask will force-feed nutrients into the skin.

Sensitive and Sensitized Skin or Rosacea

FILL IN THE BLANK

l. The primary goal when treating sensitive skin is to _____ the skin.

m. Individuals with sensitive skin should avoid stimulating, drying products and

_____.

n. A gentle cleanser, less steam and heat, an _____ peel, and a soothing alginate _____ mask are recommended products/procedures for sensitive skin.

Hyperpigmentation

FILL IN THE BLANK

o. The best preventive measures for hyperpigmentation are to _____,

_____, and _____.

p. Brighteners such as kojic acid, mulberry, licorice root, bearberry, and azaleic acid are known to

_____.

Oily Skin

FILL IN THE BLANK

q. Oily and combination skin is caused by _____ and is (thicker) in texture.

r. Oily skin is less prone to _____.

DESCRIBE ACNE FACIALS

CASE STUDY

14. Dara is an esthetician who specializes in acne facials. In fact, she has several clients who travel from other towns specifically for her treatment. Let's look in on one of Dara's appointments. Choose the word or phrase that best completes each sentence about recommended practices for acne facials.

    Dara's treatment plan for her client includes clearing the follicles by deep cleansing and extractions. However, it focuses primarily on _____.

    a. minimizing large pores

    b. cleansing the trapped oil

    c. controlling scars

    d. balancing the skin

_____ are products Dara can use on her client in different percentages to dissolve the dead skin cells and keep skin exfoliated.

a. AHAs

b. Sulfur masks

c. Enzymes

d. Benzoyl peroxide

When selecting products for home care, Dara does not choose _____ products.

a. comedogenic

b. natural

c. BHA

d. water-based

Dara uses the process of _____ to soften sebum in follicles.

a. extraction

b. toning

c. desincrustation

d. massaging the face

Dara knows that in her state, she is not legally allowed to use _____ to extract closed comedones and gently pierce the skin.

a. a comedone extractor

b. a lancet

c. cotton strips

d. gloves

Acne Treatment

LABELING

15. Label the illustrations with the correct acne pustule form.

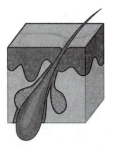 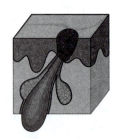 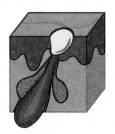 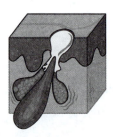 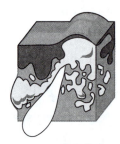

_____   _____   _____   _____   _____

SHORT ANSWER

16. Once you've labeled the illustration for how acne pustules form, explain in your own words what is occurring in the illustration from letters A to E.

_____

_____

_____

_____

_____

Products and Equipment for Acne Care

MATCHING

17. Match each product to its recommended use for acne.

a. beta hydroxy acid	d. vitamin A	g. spot blemish treatments
b. sulfur mask	e. benzoyl peroxide	h. vitamin C
c. AHA	f. kojic acid	

_____ has healing effects

_____ seeks out oil and cleanses sebum further from the skin

_____ used in different percentages to help dissolve dead skin cells

_____ brightens the skin's appearance

_____ applied only on areas after cleansing

_____ helps to reduce flaking and restores the skin's suppleness

_____ exfoliates the skin and dries blemishes

_____ releases oxygen that kills bacteria

Acne Care Tips

SHORT ANSWER

18. Tom visits the salon to seek help with his acne flare-ups. As his esthetician, give him five different tips he could try to help keep the acne under control.

_____

_____

_____

_____

_____

_____

_____

_____

_____

_____

_____

_____

_____

Extraction Techniques

MATCHING

19. Match the picture to the extraction method it is depicting. Answer options may be used more than once.

a. manual	c. comedone extractor
b. cotton swab	d. lancet

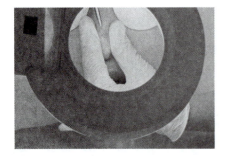 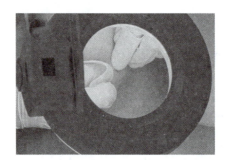 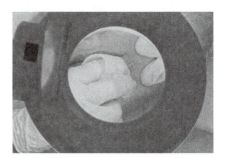

_____ _____ _____

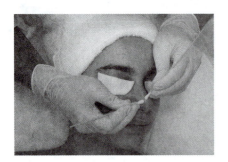 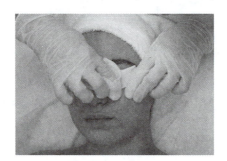 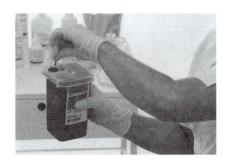

_____ _____ _____

CHAPTER 8 Facial Treatments **175**

PERFORM AN ACNE TREATMENT PROCEDURE

FILL IN THE BLANK

20. Number the following steps in the proper sequence for the acne procedure. The steps listed below are not an exact match to the chapter steps. Use your knowledge of acne treatment to put the steps in the correct order.

_____ Steam and apply serum.

_____ Wash hands and put on gloves.

_____ Apply a clay-based mask for deep cleansing. Remove the mask.

_____ Apply moisturizer.

_____ Analyze the skin.

_____ Apply astringent/toner.

_____ Perform galvanic or high-frequency treatment.

_____ Perform extractions.

_____ Proceed with desincrustation.

_____ Perform deep cleansing.

_____ Apply a soothing mask. Remove with wet cotton.

_____ Finish with the post-treatment consultation.

DISCUSS MEN'S SKIN CARE TREATMENT OPTIONS

TRUE OR FALSE

21. For the following statements on men's skin care, circle *T* if true or *F* if false. Explain your answer in the space provided.

    T   F   Professional movements during a man's facial should be in the direction opposite of hair growth.

    T   F   Men need aggressive products so they can feel the results of your services.

    T   F   Pseudofolliculitis is characterized by bumps that are filled with pus.

    T   F   A man's home care regimen should initially include only two products.

WORD REVIEW

MATCHING

22. Match the term to the correct definition.

a. express facial	c. facial	e. desincrustation
b. extraction	d. vasoconstricting	

_____   manual removal of impurities and comedones

_____   causes vascular constriction of capillaries and reduced blood flow

_____   process used to soften and emulsify sebum and comedones (blackheads) in the follicles.

_____   professional service designed to improve the appearance of the skin that takes less than 30 minutes

_____   professional service designed to improve and rejuvenate the skin

DISCOVERIES AND ACCOMPLISHMENTS

In the space below, write notes about 10 key concepts discussed in this chapter. Share your discoveries with some of the other students in your class and ask them if your notes are helpful. You may want to revise your discoveries based on good ideas shared by your peers.

Discoveries:

_____

_____

_____

_____

_____

_____

_____

_____

_____

_____

_____

_____

List at least three things you have accomplished since your last entry that relate to your career goals.

Accomplishments:

_____

_____

_____

_____

_____

_____

_____

_____

_____

_____

_____

_____

EXAM REVIEW

MULTIPLE CHOICE

1. A client wants to know why she should add a facial to her regular skin care. What can a facial provide a client beyond skin care?

    a. stress reduction

    b. fitness improvement

    c. decreased appetite

    d. increased metabolism

2. Dionne knows that her skin condition is affected by too much sun, so she wears protective clothing and sunscreen. Which of the following skin conditions does she most likely have?

    a. vitiligo

    b. hyperpigmentation

    c. hypopigmentation

    d. albinism

3. Which environmental aggravator would NOT affect acne?

    a. dirt

    b. grease

    c. humidity

    d. water

4. Zoe would like to try something new to combat her acne, especially since the prom is about one month away. Which of the following procedures, would you recommend she add to her home care twice per week?

    a. enzyme peel

    b. clay mask

    c. therapeutic sun exposure

    d. aggressive massage

5. Which of the following procedures requires you to understand the angle of the hair follicle?

    a. enzyme peels

    b. extractions

    c. clay masks

    d. product application

6. Preparation for extractions typically include all of the following except
    _____.

    a. exfoliation

    b. steaming

    c. sunscreen

    d. desincrustation

7. The skin is affected by warmth in all of the following ways except that it
    _____.

    a. softens the follicles

    b. promotes effective cleansing

    c. decreases circulation

    d. prepares skin for extractions

8. How would you describe extractions?

    a. plucking hairs with tweezers

    b. manually removing impurities and comedones from follicles

    c. reducing excess hair from nostrils with a nose trimmer

    d. chemically extracting pigment

9. When in the facial process should a calming, hydrating mask be applied?

    a. anytime

    b. at the beginning

    c. at the end

    d. never

10. Why should you offer clients water after performing services?

    a. to advertise the brand of water

    b. to upsell

    c. to increase your tip

    d. to facilitate rehydration

11. Ellie has had a difficult morning and received a speeding ticket on her way to work. As she prepares to meet her first client, which of the following should she do?

    a. Never come in to work when she is upset.

    b. Never discuss personal problems with the client.

    c. Share her problems only with clients she knows well.

    d. Discuss how to handle her problems with her clients.

12. What is NOT among the reasons clients should arrive 15 minutes prior to appointments?

    a. fill out the consultation form

    b. get into a robe

    c. help you prep the treatment room

    d. prepare for their treatment

13. When should the client be shown the area where he or she can change clothes and store any belongings?

    a. only when the client asks to see the area

    b. after completing the client consultation form

    c. at the end of the appointment

    d. immediately upon arrival in the salon

14. What should female clients be instructed to remove before a facial treatment?

    a. panties

    b. bra

    c. belt

    d. stockings

15. Who is responsible for instructing the client on how to get comfortable on the facial bed?

    a. spa assistant

    b. receptionist

    c. manager

    d. esthetician

16. When in the process of draping the hair do you place the towel on the headrest?

    a. at any time throughout the process

    b. whenever the client specifically requests you to do so

    c. at the beginning of the process

    d. after the client settles on the treatment table

17. Which of the following is an important benefit of facials to mention to clients?

    a. deep cleanse and exfoliate

    b. address conditions such as dryness or oiliness

    c. lessen the appearance of blemishes and wrinkles

    d. all of the above

18. Desiree is getting an express facial today; which step in a basic facial will you most likely skip?

    a. moisturizer

    b. extractions

    c. product application

    d. draping

19. Starr is a new student and does not understand why estheticians need to know what a client is doing for home care. What do you say to her?

    a. It is probably the least important factor in successful skin care, so you can skip asking the client about it.

    b. It is probably the most important factor in successful skin care, as it impacts what products and procedures you will use.

    c. Home care has no impact whatsoever on overall skin care, so you never ask.

    d. Very few clients perform any type of home care program, so you stopped asking years ago.

20. What should you do for about 15 minutes after the first treatment with a new client?

    a. demonstrate high-priced products

    b. explain why tips affect your income

    c. explain proper home care

    d. perform a client consultation

21. Which of the following is true of an express facial?

    a. has fewer steps than a basic facial

    b. has more steps than a basic facial

    c. is the same as a basic facial with less time spent on each step

    d. has no treatment benefits because less time is spent on each step

22. There are many variations of a basic facial. What should you tell a client who wants to know the approximate length of a full, basic facial?

    a. 10 minutes

    b. 25 minutes

    c. 45 minutes

    d. 60 minutes

23. What skin type is associated with the treatment goal of stimulating sebum production?
    a. oily skin
    b. couperose skin
    c. dry skin
    d. damaged skin

24. A client has very dry skin. What type of enzyme peel should you use to exfoliate during treatment?
    a. gentle
    b. medium
    c. harsh
    d. enzyme peels should not be used on dry skin

25. What is NOT a recommended treatment for dry skin?
    a. moisturizing cream with an oil base
    b. antioxidants
    c. sunscreen finish
    d. harsh exfoliation

26. What can be caused by smoking, extreme weight loss, and physiological disease?
    a. hypopigmentation
    b. accelerated skin aging
    c. couperose skin
    d. albinism

27. What do facial treatments offer in addition to relaxation?
    a. changes in skin type
    b. improvement of the skin's health
    c. weight loss
    d. stimulated hair growth

28. What is true of facial treatments?
    a. they are the core treatments that estheticians perform
    b. they are minor elements of the services performed by estheticians
    c. only clients with damaged skin truly benefit from facial treatments
    d. clients with damaged skin are beyond the help of facial treatments

29. Jack is considering having a facial but isn't clear on what a facial treatment involves. Which of the following best describes a facial?

    a. professional service designed to improve and rejuvenate the skin

    b. application of makeup to make the client's face more attractive

    c. medical procedure involving the use of injected chemicals

    d. surgical procedure more commonly known as a face lift

30. A client thinks they may need a prescription for acne care. Who can issue prescriptions?

    a. receptionists

    b. physicians

    c. estheticians

    d. salon managers

31. Jolene likes to stay current on trends in the esthetic industry. How often should she take a class or go to a conference?

    a. at least once a month

    b. at least once a year

    c. every two years

    d. every five years

32. The manager of a spa emphasizes that estheticians need to speak to clients in a quiet and professional manner. Why is this helpful?

    a. Clients will believe everything you say.

    b. Clients will take all of your advice.

    c. Clients will relax and enjoy their treatment.

    d. Clients will be able to sleep if needed.

33. Disposable cotton to remove facial masks can be referred to as _____.

    a. cotton balls

    b. cotton compress

    c. cotton swabs

    d. astringent

34. Which of the following is NOT a reason to remove jewelry before performing services?

    a. Jewelry might clash with your uniform.

    b. Jewelry might injure or scratch the client.

    c. Jewelry might cause a distraction during the service.

    d. Jewelry might inhibit your movements during the service.

35. A client is in a rush and can't stay for a full facial. You advise a mini-facial because its length is only _____.

    a. 5 minutes

    b. 10 minutes

    c. 30 minutes

    d. 40 minutes

36. In a men's skin care treatment, what should you do after cleansing the client's skin?

    a. show the client where to change into a robe for the service

    b. complete a thorough skin analysis with a magnifying lamp

    c. perform a client consultation to identify which services to perform

    d. get the client comfortable on the treatment table

37. If permitted in your state, lancets are used for all of the following except _____.

    a. nodules

    b. pimples

    c. comedones

    d. pustules

38. When during the facial procedure should you apply moisturizer and/or sunscreen?

    a. at the beginning

    b. in the middle

    c. at the end

    d. anytime

39. Jean notices that a male client has folliculitis. How will she explain it to him? Folliculitis is _____.

    a. excessive hair around the face

    b. when goose bumps are present

    c. an abnormally low number of hair follicles

    d. an inflammation of the hair follicles

40. What is the common name for pseudofolliculitis?

    a. goose bumps

    b. razor bumps

    c. wind burn

    d. sunburn

41. What causes pseudofolliculitis?
    a. use of hair dye
    b. improper shaving
    c. use of Rogaine®
    d. poor sleep habits

42. Why should comedogenic products be avoided for clients with acne?
    a. These products are typically water based.
    b. Clients with acne experience pain from comedogenic products.
    c. Clients with acne bleed easily after exposure to comedogenic products.
    d. These products tend to aggravate or produce acne symptoms.

43. During an acne treatment, why is it important to soften the outmost layer of the skin prior to beginning any extraction?
    a. because the skin may be tight and dehydrated
    b. because the skin may be oily and loose
    c. because the skin may be firm and dry
    d. because the skin may be thin and elastic

44. Astringent application is critical after extractions for all of the following reasons except _____.
    a. rehydrating the skin
    b. reducing secondary infections
    c. cleansing the skin
    d. removing redness

45. All of the following are important considerations for a men's skin care product line except for _____.
    a. basic
    b. heavy lotions
    c. simple routine
    d. light fragrance

Client Intake Form and Medical History

In order to provide you with the most appropriate treatment, we need you to complete the following questionnaire. All information is confidential.

Date _____

Name _____ **Date of birth** (optional) _____
(please print)

Email address _____

Address _____ _____ _____ _____
Street   City   State   Zip

Phone number (easiest number to reach you) _____

Occupation _____

How were you referred to us? _____

MEDICAL HISTORY

Are you currently under the care of a physician for any reason? _____ ☐ Yes   ☐ No

If yes, for what? _____

History	Yes	No	Date/List/Comments
List all medications, supplements, and vitamins			
List allergies			
Accutane			
Antibiotics			
Birth control pills			
Hormones			
Aspirin, ibuprofen use			
Retin-A®, Tretinoin			
Metrogel®, MetroCream®			
Glycolic acid on a regular basis			
Antidepressants			
Sun reactions			
Medication allergies			
Food allergies			
Aspirin allergy			
Latex allergy			
Lidocaine allergy			
Hydrocortisone allergy			

(Continued)

History	Yes	No	Date/List/Comments
Diabetes			
Smoking history			
Cold sores, herpes			
Bleeding disorders			
Autoimmune, HIV			
Pregnant or planning to be			
Pacemaker			
Implants of any kind: Dental, breast, facial			
Migraine headaches			
Glaucoma			
Cancer			
Arthritis			
Hepatitis			
Thyroid imbalance			
Seizure disorder			
Active infection			
Radiation in last three months			
Skin Conditions			
Acne			
Melasma			
Tattoos, perm makeup, and microblading			
Vitiligo			
Keloid scarring			
Skin/laser treatments at another office			If so, when? Results
Botox			If so, when? Results
Fillers			If so, when? Results
Hair removal			If so, when? Results
Chemical peels			If so, when? Results
Sun exposure/tanning bed in last week? Self tanner?			If so, when? Results
List Medical Issues Not Listed Above			

(Continued)

CURRENT SKIN CARE AND LIFESTYLE

1. How do you wash your face?   ☐ Soap   ☐ Cleanser

2. If soap, what brand? _____

3. If cleanser, what brand name? _____

4. Do you use a moisturizer?   ☐ Yes   ☐ No

5. Are you on a special diet?   ☐ Yes   ☐ No

   If yes, please specify. _____

6. Do you consume water daily?   ☐ Yes   ☐ No

   If yes, how much? _____

7. Do you drink coffee, tea, or soda daily?   ☐ Yes   ☐ No

   Coffee ounces _____ Tea ounces _____ Soda ounces _____

8. Do you exercise?   ☐ Yes   ☐ No

   If yes, how often? _____

9. Have you ever had a facial?   ☐ Yes   ☐ No

   If yes, when was your last facial? _____

10. Do you give yourself facials at home?   ☐ Yes   ☐ No

    If yes, how often? _____

11. List additional cosmetics and skin care products you are currently using:

What is the primary reason for your visit today? (Select all that apply in the list below.)
☐   I'm concerned about facial or body hair and would like information on ways to get rid of it.
☐   I'm concerned about fine lines around my eyes.
☐   I'm concerned about scowl lines when I frown.
☐   I'm concerned about pigmentation or age spots.
☐   I'm concerned about broken capillaries on my face or spider veins on my legs.
☐   I'm concerned about skin laxity and sagging.
☐   I'm concerned about the lines around my mouth.
☐   I'd like more defined lips.
☐   Other (please list skin concerns below)

I certify that the preceding medical, personal, and skin history statements are true and correct. I am aware that it is my responsibility to inform the technician of my current medical and health conditions and to update this information at subsequent visits. A current history is essential for the provider to execute appropriate treatment procedures. I have signed the consent form for this procedure. I had the opportunity to ask questions prior to the treatment. I accept arbitration as a means of resolution for practice liability.

_____   _____
Client Signature   Date

PROCEDURE 8–1: PRE-SERVICE: PREPARING THE CLIENT FOR TREATMENT

Evaluate your practical skills.

CRITERIA	COMPETENT	NEEDS WORK	IMPROVEMENT PLAN
Preparation			
Perform Procedure 7–1: Pre-Service—Preparing the Treatment Room to set up the treatment room and supplies.			
Procedure			
1. Greet the client in the reception area with a warm smile and in a professional manner. Introduce yourself if you've never met, make eye contact, and shake hands. Be sure your handshake is firm and sincere.			
2. Discuss the completed client intake form with the client and confirm their service. Ask about any client concerns and set the expectations for today's service.			
3. Ensure there are no contraindications for the treatment scheduled. Have your client sign a consent form before every service.			
4. Escort the client to the dressing area or the treatment room to change. Inform the client where to place personal items. Ask the client to remove all jewelry and place in a sealable plastic bag to secure items. Due to liability issues do not handle the client's jewelry. Have the client remove contact lenses as well (optional, if wearing them).			
5. Provide them with a robe, spa wrap, and slippers. Explain which clothing may need to be removed and show them how to put on the spa wrap. Indicate where to go once they have changed. Then allow them to undress privately. Always knock before re-entering the room.			
6. Depending on the service to be performed, instruct the client to lie either face down or face up on the treatment table or to take a seat in the treatment chair.			
7. Place a bolster under the bottom sheet, below their knees, to relieve pressure on the lower back if they are facing up. (This alleviates pressure on the lower back.) If your client is facing down, place a rolled towel or small bolster under their ankles.			
8. Bring the second sheet up and blanket across the décolleté. Then place a hand towel across the chest on top of the covers.			

9. Secure a disposable headband, towel, or other head covering around the client's head to protect the hair, making sure all the hair is off the face. To drape the head with a towel, follow steps a, b, and c. a. During setup in Procedure 7–1, you placed a hand towel on the headrest. Fold the towel into a triangle from one of the top corners to the opposite lower corner, and place it over the headrest with the fold facing down. b. When the client is in a reclined position, the back of the head should rest on the towel, so that the sides of the towel can be brought up to the center of the forehead to cover the hairline. c. Use a disposable headband to hold the towel in place. Use a spatula or the edge of your finger to make sure that all strands of hair are tucked under the towel, that the earlobes are not bent, and that the towel is not wrapped too tightly.			
10. Wash your hands with soap and warm water as detailed in Procedure 5–3: Proper Hand Washing located in Milady Standard Foundations. Always wash your hands and put on gloves before starting any treatment.			
11. Proceed with the next steps in your facial treatment.			

PROCEDURE 8–2: REMOVE EYE MAKEUP AND LIPSTICK

Evaluate your practical skills.

CRITERIA	COMPETENT	NEEDS WORK	IMPROVEMENT PLAN
Preparation			
Perform Procedure 7–1: Pre-Service—Preparing the Treatment Room and Procedure 8–1: Pre-Service—Preparing the Client for Treatment.			
Procedure			
A. Eye Makeup Removal			
Note: If the client is wearing contacts, do not remove the eye makeup. Be especially gentle when cleansing the eyes because the skin around the eyes is very sensitive and can become irritated. Do not get cleanser into the eyes.			
1. Saturate two cotton rounds with a mild cleanser (usually a pH of 7.0–7.2 is recommended) or makeup remover. You also have the choice of using gloved hands to apply the cleanser.			

2. Ask the client to close their eyes. Start with the client's left eye. With one hand, gently raise and hold the client's eyebrow. With the cotton pad in your other hand, gently wipe across the top of the eyelid from the nose outward. Use downward movements with the cleansing pad to cleanse the eyelid and lashes. Gently rinse with cotton or gauze pads.			
3. While cleansing the eyes, rotate the pad to provide a clean, unused surface. Repeat step 2 as necessary to remove eye makeup.			
4. Wipe under the eyes, sweeping in toward the nose. Remove any makeup underneath the eyes and along the lash line with a cotton swab or pad. Place the edge of the pad under the lower lashes at the outside corner of the eye, and slide the pad toward the inner corner of the eye. The mascara will gradually work loose and can be wiped clean. Always be gentle around the eyes; never rub or stretch the skin, as it is very delicate and thin.			
5. Make a complete circular pattern around the eye. Use the pad or a cotton swab to wipe inward under the eye toward the nose and then outward over the top of the eyelid.			
6. Rinse the eye area with a pad or cotton rounds soaked (not dripping) in warm water to remove the eye makeup remover. Make sure the remover is rinsed off thoroughly.			
B. Lipstick Removal			
7. To remove the majority of the lipstick, first support the lip and wipe away the lipstick using a dry tissue, then discard the tissue.			
8. Then, apply cleanser to a gauze or cotton pad. With your left hand, hold taut the left side of the client's mouth. Wipe from the corner to the center to prevent the lipstick from being wiped out onto the skin surrounding the mouth.			
9. Repeat the procedure on the other side until the lips are clean. Proceed with the next step of the basic facial.			

PROCEDURE 8–3: APPLYING A CLEANSING PRODUCT

Evaluate your practical skills.

CRITERIA	COMPETENT	NEEDS WORK	IMPROVEMENT PLAN
Preparation			
Perform Procedure 7–1: Pre-Service—Preparing the Treatment Room and Procedure 8–1: Pre-Service—Preparing the Client for Treatment.			
Procedure			
1. Apply warm towels (optional). Check the temperature and apply one towel to the décolleté and one to the face. Leave on for at least 1 minute and then remove.			
2. Choose a cleanser appropriate to the client's skin type. Use a spatula to remove the product from the container unless using a squirt or pump bottle. Apply approximately one teaspoon of the product to the fingers or palms of the hand and spread evenly between your gloved hands and fingertips.			
3. Use circular motions to distribute the product onto the fingertips. You are now ready to apply the product to the client's décolleté, neck, and face. Cleanse each area using six passes. If starting on the décolleté, start in the center and work out to the sides moving up to the neck. Be guided by your instructor.			
4. Start applying a small amount of the product by placing both hands, palms down, on the neck. Slide hands back toward the ears until the pads of the fingers rest at a point directly beneath the earlobes. While applying the product, it is suggested that hands are not lifted from the client's face until you are finished.			
5. Reverse the hands, with the backs of the fingers now resting on the skin, and slide the fingers along the jawline to the chin.			
6. Reverse the hands again, and slide the fingers back over the cheeks and center of the face until the pads of the fingers come to rest directly in front of the ears.			
7. Reverse the hands again, and slide the fingers forward over the cheekbones to the nose. Cleanse the upper lip area under the nose with sideways strokes from the center area moving outward. Then slide up to the sides of the nose.			
8. With the pads of the middle fingers, make small, circular motions on the top of the nose and on each side of the nose. Avoid pushing the product into the nose.			

	COMPETENT	NEEDS WORK	IMPROVEMENT PLAN
9. Slide the fingers up to the forehead and outward toward the temples, pausing with a slight pressure on the temples. Slide fingers across the forehead using circles or long strokes from side to side. Slowly lift your hands off the client's face.			
10. Proceed to Procedure 8–4: Removing Products if the product used needs to be removed, for example, a cleanser or massage cream.			

PROCEDURE 8–4: REMOVING PRODUCTS

Evaluate your practical skills.

CRITERIA	COMPETENT	NEEDS WORK	IMPROVEMENT PLAN
Procedure			
1. Starting at the décolleté, cleanse sideways and up to the neck. When removing the cleanser, mask, or exfoliant, you should make three passes or however many are necessary until no residual makeup shows.			
2. Cleanse the neck using upward strokes. To keep the pad from slipping from the hand, pinch the edge of the pad between the thumb and upper part of the forefinger. It is important that most of the surface of the pad remain in contact with the skin. Do not exert pressure on the Adam's apple in the center of the neck.			
3. Starting directly under the chin, slide along the jawline, stopping directly under the ear. Repeat the movement on the other side of the face. Alternate back and forth three times on each side of the face, or do the movement concurrently by using both hands at the same time.			
4. Starting at the jawline, use upward movements to cleanse the cheeks.			
5. Continue the upward movement and cross over the chin to the other cheek if you are using only one hand.			
6. Continue the cleansing movement with approximately six strokes on each cheek.			
7. Under the eyes, use inward motions to avoid tugging at the eye area.			
8. Cleanse the area directly underneath the nose by using downward and sideways strokes. Start at the center and work outward toward the corners of the mouth. Rinse at least three times on each side of the face.			

	COMPETENT	NEEDS WORK	IMPROVEMENT PLAN
9. Starting on the bridge of the nose, cleanse the sides of the nose and the area directly next to it. Use light, outward movements.			
10. Starting at the center of the forehead, move outward to the temples. Apply a slight pressure on the pressure points of the temples. Repeat the movement three times on each side of the forehead.			
11. Check the face to make sure there is no residue left on the skin. Feather over the areas of the face with the fingertips to check that it is well rinsed. Discard all used supplies in the trash can.			
12. Cover the client's eyes with eye pads and prepare to perform the skin analysis.			

PROCEDURE 8–5: PERFORMING THE BASIC FACIAL

Evaluate your practical skills.

CRITERIA	COMPETENT	NEEDS WORK	IMPROVEMENT PLAN
Preparation			
Perform Procedure 7–1: Pre-Service—Preparing the Treatment Room and Procedure 8–1: Pre-Service—Preparing the Client for Treatment.			
Preheat the steamer ahead of time. Check that the water level is at the appropriate fill line.			
Procedure			
1. Wash your hands and apply gloves.			
2. Apply warm towels (optional step). After checking the temperature, apply one towel to the décolleté and one to the face. a. Hold the ends of the towels with both hands on either side of the face. Lay the center of the towel on the chin and drape each side across the face with the towel edges draped over to the opposite corner across the forehead. b. To remove, lift each end and remove. For product removal: Use the towels over the hands as mitts. Be guided by your instructor on this method.			
3. Remove eye makeup and lipstick. As learned in Procedure 8–2, remember to ask about contact lenses before putting product on the eyes. If the client is wearing contacts, do not remove the eye makeup.			

4. Perform facial cleansing (steps 4 to 10). Remove about one-half to one teaspoon of cleanser from the container (with a clean spatula if it is not a squirt-top or pump-type lid). Place it on the fingertips or in the palm and then apply a small amount to your gloved fingertips. This conserves the amount of product you use.			
5. Starting at the neck or décolleté and with a sweeping movement, use both hands to spread the cleanser upward and outward on the chin, jaws, cheeks, and temples.			
6. Spread the cleanser down the nose and along its sides and bridge. Continue to the upper lip area. Cleanse the upper lip area under the nose with sideways strokes from the center area moving outward.			
7. Make small, circular movements with the fingertips around the nostrils and sides of the nose. Continue with upward-sweeping movements between the brows and across the forehead to the temples.			
8. Apply more cleanser to the neck and chest with long, outward strokes. Cleanse the area in small, circular motions from the center of the chest and neck toward the outside, moving upward. Try to use both hands at the same time on each side when applying or removing product.			
9. Visually divide the face into left and right halves from the center. Continue moving upward with circular motions on the face from the chin and cheeks, and up toward the forehead using both hands, one on each side.			
10. Starting at the center of the forehead, continue with the circular pattern out to the temples. Move the fingertips lightly in a circle around the eyes to the temples and then back to the center of the forehead. Lift your hands slowly off of the face when you finish cleansing.			
11. Remove the cleanser. Start at the neck or forehead and follow the contours of the face. Move up or down the face in a consistent pattern, depending on where you start, according to the instructor's procedures. Remove all the cleanser from one area of the face before proceeding to the next. (Under the nostrils, use downward strokes when applying or removing products to avoid pushing product up the nose. This is uncomfortable and will make the client tense.)			
12. Make sure there is no residue left on the skin. Blot your hands on a clean towel, and touch the face with dry fingertips to check.			
13. Analyze the skin (steps 13 to 15). Cover the client's eyes with eye pads. Try not to cover what you need to look at around the eyes.			

14. Position the magnifying light where you want it before starting the facial, so that you can easily maneuver it over the face. Turn on the lamp away from client before lining it up over the face.			
15. Note the skin type and condition, sensitivity, hydration, elasticity, and feel the texture of the skin. Remember to look, touch, ask and listen.			
16. Cleanse the face again (optional). Some treatment protocols do not include this second cleansing. Be guided by your instructor.			
17. Exfoliation (optional). If exfoliation is part of the service, it could be done at this time while steaming. Tone after removing exfoliant to rebalance pH of the skin.			
18. Massage the face (steps 18 to 22). Use the facial manipulations described in Chapter 9, Facial Massage. Select a water-soluble massage cream or product appropriate to the client's skin type.			
19. Use the same procedure as you did for product application to apply the massage cream to the face, neck, shoulders, and chest. Apply the warmed product in long, slow strokes with fingers or a soft fan brush, moving in a set pattern.			
20. Perform the massage as directed.			
21. Remove the massage medium. Use warm towels or 4" × 4" esthetics wipes and follow the same procedure as for removing other products or cleanser.			
22. Steam the face using the steamer (steps 22 and 23). Skip to step 24 if using towels. The steamer should be preheated at the start of the facial. Wait for it to start steaming, and then turn on the second ozone button if applicable while steaming. (Remember that steam should be avoided on sensitive skin types.)			
23. Check to make sure the steamer is not too close to the client (it should be approximately 18 inches away) and that it is steaming the face evenly. If you hold your hands close to the sides of the client's face, you can feel if the steam is reaching both sides of the face. Steam for approximately 5 to 10 minutes. Turn off the steamer immediately after use.			
24. Steam the face using towels. If using towels in place of steam, remember to test them for the correct temperature. Ask the client if they are comfortable with the temperature. Towels are left on for approximately 2 minutes or until they begin to cool. Steam or warm towels should be used carefully on couperose skin.			

25. Perform extractions (if needed). Extractions are done immediately after the steam, while the skin is still warm. Refer to the extractions section of this chapter to incorporate this step into your basic facial procedure if it is applicable to your facility.			
26. Apply a mask (steps 26 to 29). Choose a mask formulated for the client's skin condition. Remove the mask from its container, and place it in the palm or a small mixing bowl. (Use a clean spatula or brush, if necessary, to prevent cross-contamination.) Warming the mask is recommended for better results as well as the client's comfort.			
27. Apply the mask with a brush or spatula, usually starting at the neck. Use long, slow strokes from the center of the face, moving outward to the sides.			
28. Proceed to the jawline and apply the mask on the face from the center outward. Avoid the eye area unless the mask is appropriate for that area.			
29. Allow the mask to remain on the face for approximately 7 to 10 minutes.			
30. Remove the mask. Use warm moist towels or 4" × 4" esthetics wipes for removal. Cream-based masks can be wiped off, while clay masks can be removed with a mummy-style mask. Some masks may peel off, such as alginate or sheet masks.			
31. Apply the toner. Apply the toner product appropriate for the client's skin type.			
32. Apply serums, as well as eye and lip treatments. Serums as well as eye and lip creams are optional for application before the final moisturizer.			
33. Apply a moisturizer (and an additional sunscreen as appropriate).			
34. Postconsultation and home care. End the facial by removing your gloves, and quietly letting the client know you are finished. Give the client instructions for getting dressed. Have the client come out to the reception area when they are ready to discuss the home care products and regimen.			
Post-Service			
Complete Procedure 8–9: Post-Service Procedure and Procedure 7–2: Post-Service—Clean-Up and Preparation for the Next Client, including advising the client, promoting products, scheduling a next appointment, thanking the client, and cleaning and setting up the treatment room.			

PROCEDURE 8–6: APPLYING AND REMOVING THE COTTON COMPRESS

Evaluate your practical skills.

CRITERIA	COMPETENT	NEEDS WORK	IMPROVEMENT PLAN
Procedure			
1. After the mask or product has set for the appropriate time, take one cotton 4" × 4" square, open to 4" × 8", and saturate with water.			
2. After squeezing out excess water, place the cotton lengthwise, first covering the neck.			
3. Saturate a second piece of cotton with water and make a small opening for the mouth. Place across the chin and mouth from one side of the mandible to the other just below the nose.			
4. When placing the third piece of cotton over the bridge of the nose and across the eyes, be sure to leave the nostrils exposed and airways open.			
5. Place the fourth piece of wet cotton across the forehead, covering from temple to temple and cheek to cheek from one zygomatic bone to the other. Keep the cotton moist to help "loosen" mask for flawless removal, but not soaking wet to avoid dripping down the client's neck.			
6. To remove the mummy mask, starting at the forehead, use a flat hand to wipe the product from one side of the face to the other. If you are right-handed, remove from left to right; if left-handed, right to left.			
7. Fold the cotton under as you are removing the mask, as this will pick up more of the product and assist in quicker and cleaner removal.			
8. Repeat the same movement on the cheek and mandible area. Finish removing from your client's cheek and nose area.			
9. Remove the product and cotton from the neck. Use more cotton to remove any remaining residue.			
10. Once residue is removed, refresh skin with hydrating mist or the appropriate toner/astringent, and then blot with tissue.			

PROCEDURE 8–7: PERFORMING EXTRACTIONS

Evaluate your practical skills.

CRITERIA	COMPETENT	NEEDS WORK	IMPROVEMENT PLAN
Preparing Premade Pads			
If you are using 4" × 4" or 2" × 2" premade pads, apply astringent to pads (without oversaturating them) and wrap around your fingers. Always wear gloves during extractions and during the entire facial treatment.			
Preparing for Extractions			
Extractions must be performed in such a way as to not cause further damage to the skin or make the acne worse.			
1. Wash hands and put on a new pair of gloves. Gloves are critical here because this is an invasive procedure.			
2. Place eye pads over the client's eyes.			
3. Position the magnifying lamp over the client's face. Always look through a magnifying lamp when performing extractions. This will protect you from any debris that come from the clogged pore. Again, advanced acne such as cysts and nodules should be treated only by a dermatologist.			
4. Proceed with manual comedone removal, using the cotton swab technique, comedone extractor, or a lancet as permitted by your state board regulations.			
A. Manually Removing Comedones			
1. Wrap your fingers with cotton or gauze slightly moistened with a few drops of astringent at the tips.			
2. For proper removal of comedones, use the side of your fingertips to exert firm pressure on the skin surrounding the blackhead or comedone, applying slight pressure from side to side, alternating angles to gently lift the comedone from the follicle opening. Comedone extractors can also be used for this (be guided by your instructor). Do not squeeze with your nail, only the side of your finger.			
3. Start at the chin. On a flat area, press down, under, in, and up. Work around the plug, pressing down, in, and up. Bring fingers in toward each other around the follicle without pinching. Place the comedone on a tissue and proceed to other areas.			

4. Nose. Slide fingers down each side of the nose, holding the nostril tissue firmly, but do not press down too firmly on the nose. The fingers on top do the sliding, while the other one holds close to the bottom of the follicle. Do not cut off the air flow to the nostrils.			
5. Cheeks. Slide fingers together down the cheek, holding each section of the skin as you go. The lower hand holds and the other hand slides toward the lower hand.			
6. Forehead; upper cheekbones. Extract as on the chin: press down, in, and up.			
7. Dispose of gloves and supplies properly. Change gloves to continue the facial treatment.			
B. Using the Cotton Swab Technique			
1. Hold the cotton swabs with your index finger and thumb and gently press down on both sides of the follicle.			
2. If the contents do not expel right away, move the swabs from side to side and the debris will gently lift up. Do not apply too much pressure, as it can bruise the client's skin. In both cases, if the contents are still not expelling, simply leave the comedone for the next treatment, and proceed to the next area of concern.			
C. Comedone Extractor			
1. To use the comedone extractor, place the loop over the lesion so that the lesion is inside the loop.			
2. Press gently next to the lesion to push it up and out. Be aware that the pressure exerted can traumatize tissues. The follicle walls can rupture, spilling sebum and bacteria into the dermis. This debris can cause infection and irritation that leads to the start of even more blemishes.			
D. Extracting with Lancets			
1. Wrap the index fingers with cotton or use sterile cotton swabs.			
2. Hold the lancet parallel to the surface of the skin or at a 35-degee angle and gently pierce the skin horizontally to release sebum. If you prick into the skin in a downward motion, you can cause scarring.			
3. After piercing the skin horizontally, gently press down on both sides of the milia and remove it.			
4. Dispose of the lancet in the biohazard containers also known as sharps boxes. Do not reuse the lancet.			

PROCEDURE 8–8: APPLYING A SHEET MASK

Evaluate your practical skills.

CRITERIA	COMPETENT	NEEDS WORK	IMPROVEMENT PLAN
Procedure			
1. Apply the serum of your choice. (This is optional, as you may choose to just apply the sheet mask directly to the face.)			
2. With a new pair of gloves, open the sheet mask packet and place the open packet on your station.			
3. Beginning at the chin, remove the backing on the sheet mask. Apply the sheet mask in a uniform format, smoothing the mask onto the face such that the mask is optionally positioned to ensure all areas of the face are benefiting from the sheet mask.			
4. Process the mask according to the manufacturer's recommended processing time.			
5. Remove the mask and proceed with the next steps in your facial treatment.			

PROCEDURE 8–9: POST-SERVICE PROCEDURE

Evaluate your practical skills.

CRITERIA	COMPETENT	NEEDS WORK	IMPROVEMENT PLAN
A. Advising Clients and Promoting Products			
1. Before the client leaves your treatment area, ask them how they feel and if they enjoyed the service. Explain the conditions of their skin and your ideas about how to improve them. Be sure to ask if they have any questions or anything else they'd like to discuss. Be receptive and listen. Never be defensive. Determine a plan for future visits. Give the client ideas to think over for the next visit.			
2. Advise the client about proper home care and explain how the recommended professional products will help to improve any skin conditions that are present. This is the time to discuss your retail product recommendations. Explain that these products are important and how to use them.			

3. Escort the client to the reception desk and write up a service ticket for the client that includes the service provided, recommended home care, and the next visit/service that needs to be scheduled. Place all recommended home care products on the counter for the client. Review the service ticket and the product recommendations with your client.			
4. After the client has paid for their service and home care products, ask if you can schedule their next appointment. Set up the date, time, and type of service for this next appointment, write the information on your business card, and give the card to the client.			
5. Thank the client for the opportunity to work with them. Express an interest in working with them in the future. Invite the client to contact you should they have any questions or concerns about the service provided. If the client seems apprehensive, offer to call them in a day or two in order to check in with them about any issues they may have. Genuinely wish them well, shake hands, and wish them a great day.			
6. Be sure to record service information, observations, and product recommendations on the client record, and be sure you return it to the proper place for filing.			
7. Continue with setting up for the next service or end-of-day checklist as outlined in Procedure 7–2: Post-Service—Clean-Up and Preparation for the Next Client.			

EXPLAIN THE IMPORTANCE OF FACIAL MASSAGE AS AN ESTHETIC SERVICE

SHORT ANSWER

1. Give a detailed definition of massage. Then, give two reasons that facial massage is an important part of esthetic service.

_____
_____
_____
_____
_____
_____
_____

DESCRIBE THE BENEFITS OF MASSAGE

SHORT ANSWER

2. A friend says she is considering getting a massage, but is wondering if massage has any benefits. List five benefits you can tell her about.

- _____
- _____
- _____
- _____
- _____

DISCUSS FACIAL MASSAGE CONTRAINDICATIONS

SHORT ANSWER

3. Your client has a contraindication for a facial massage. What can you do if your client cannot have a facial massage?

_____

_____

_____

_____

_____

Know Your Scope of Practice

SHORT ANSWER

4. Research your state regulations and identify what areas you are allowed to massage.

_____

_____

_____

_____

_____

DESCRIBE THE FIVE TYPES OF MASSAGE MOVEMENTS USED BY ESTHETICIANS

MATCHING

5. Match the type of massage to its characteristic. The types of massage will be used more than once.

| a. effleurage | c. tapotement | e. vibration |
| b. pétrissage | d. friction | |

_____ known as percussion

_____ used to begin and end massage sessions

_____ includes kneading, squeezing, and pinching

_____ invigorating rubbing technique that stimulates circulation

_____ most stimulating form of massage

_____ slightly curve the fingers with the cushions of the fingertips touching the skin

_____ rapid shaking movement in which the esthetician uses their body and shoulders

_____ sometimes referred to as a piano movement

_____ most important of the five movements

_____ highly stimulating and should be used sparingly

_____ performed on fleshier parts of the face, shoulders, back, and arms

_____ can stimulate underlying tissues and activate circulation

_____ purifies the system by releasing carbon dioxide and other waste materials

_____ performed in a circular manner or a crisscross manner with fingers working in opposition to each other

Alternative Massage Techniques

FILL IN THE BLANK

6. Aromatherapy massage uses _____ mixed with an emulsion or oil and applied to the skin during massage movements.

7. _____ uses points to relax and balance the body.

8. _____ is a light touch that may reduce swelling and detoxify waste materials from the body.

9. _____ is a massage technique derived from Chinese medicine to release muscle tension, restore balance, and stimulate _chi_.

10. Using light inward pressure at each point and then lifting the pressure is necessary to perform _____ massage correctly.

EXPLAIN HOW TO INCORPORATE MASSAGE DURING THE FACIAL TREATMENT

SHORT ANSWER

11. Johanna asks for a facial massage during her facial treatment. How will you incorporate massage into Johanna's treatment?

_____

_____

_____

_____

_____

Learn the Technical Skills

SHORT ANSWER

12. Facial massage requires specific techniques. List five techniques you will use to perform an effective and safe facial massage.

- _____
  _____
  _____

- _____
  _____
  _____

- _____
  _____
  _____

- _____
  _____
  _____

- _____
  _____
  _____

Maintain Hand Mobility

SHORT ANSWER

13. Describe how you will maintain your hands and hand mobility.

_____
_____
_____
_____
_____

Use Proper Massage Products

SHORT ANSWER

14. What factors need to be considered when choosing a massage product?

_____

_____

_____

_____

_____

_____

Relax

SHORT ANSWER

15. Kenisha is preparing to provide a massage for a new client. What strategies should she use to prepare to give the best service possible?

- _____
- _____
- _____
- _____

Choose Your Starting Point

SHORT ANSWER

16. Anna is preparing to perform a facial massage. Where should she start the massage, and what guidelines should she use to perform the facial massage effectively?

_____

_____

_____

_____

_____

_____

Maintain Contact and Massage from Insertion to Origin

FILL IN THE BLANK

17. The _____ is where the muscle attaches to the non-moving bone.

18. Should it become necessary to lift the hands from the client's face, slow down the movement and then gently replace it with finishing movements often called _____.

19. _____ strokes can cause premature folds and wrinkles.

20. The _____ is where the muscle attaches to the bone that moves when the muscle contracts.

Check Pressure

SHORT ANSWER

21. Your next client tells you she was disappointed in her last facial massage at another salon. She says the technician did not apply enough pressure to her face. Explain to your client the reasons why you will not use much pressure either.

_____

_____

_____

_____

_____

Sharpen Your Professionalism

SHORT ANSWER

22. Clients are not always pleased with their facial treatments. List five of the main complaints that clients have about their treatments.

- _____
  _____
- _____
  _____
- _____
  _____
- _____
  _____
- _____
  _____

PERFORM A BASIC FACIAL MASSAGE

LABELING

23. Label each of the techniques of the facial massage routine in the space provided in your own words. The first step is provided for you. Write the steps for the facial routine with short explanations to help you learn the routine. Use the correct terms for the massage techniques in your explanation, such as petrissage, effleurage, vibration, tapotement, and friction.

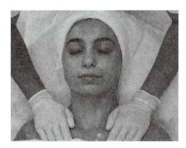 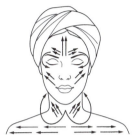

1. Start with hands on the décolleté

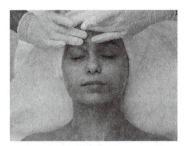 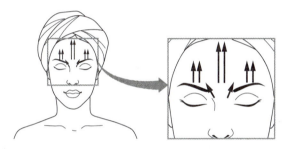

2. _____

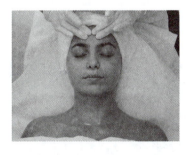 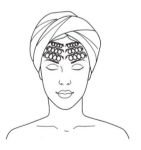

3. _____

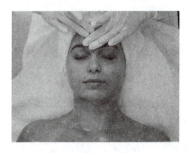 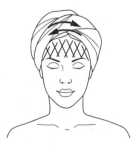

4. _____

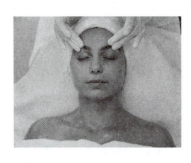
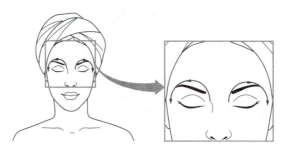

5. _____

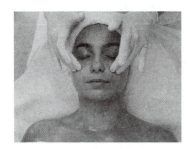
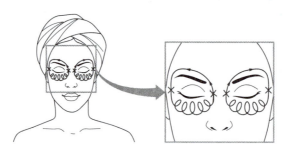

6. _____

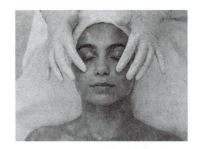
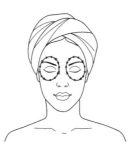

7. _____

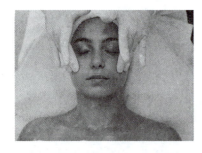
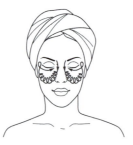

8. _____

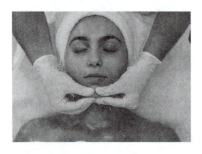
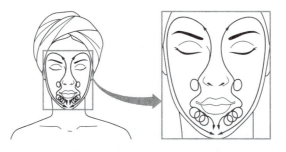

9. _____

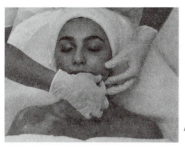 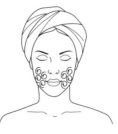 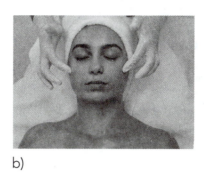 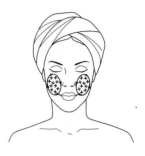

a)

b)

10a. _____   10b. _____

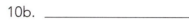

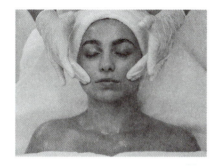 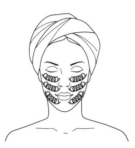

11. _____

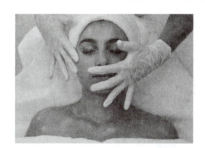 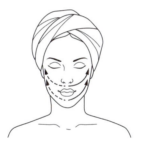

12. _____

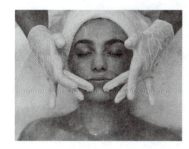 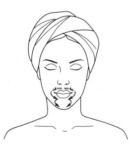

13. _____

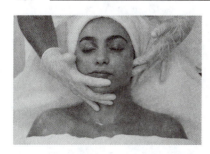 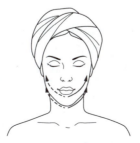

14. _____

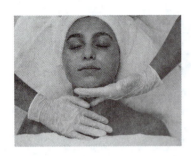
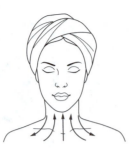

15. _____

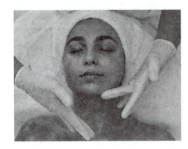
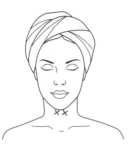

16. _____

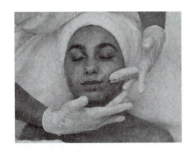
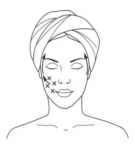

17. _____

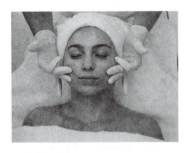
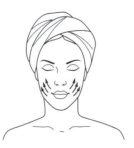

18. _____

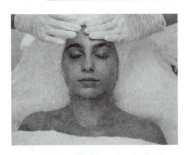
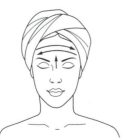

19. _____

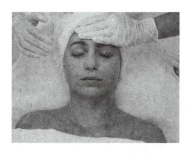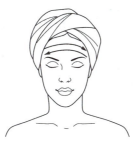

20. _____

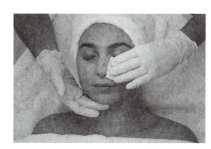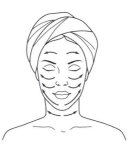

21. _____

WORD REVIEW

MATCHING

24. Match the word to its definition.

a. effleurage	d. massage	g. vibration
b. friction	e. pétrissage	
c. manual lymph drainage	f. tapotement	

_____ invigorating rubbing technique requiring pressure on the skin with the fingers or palm while moving them under an underlying structure

_____ manual or mechanical manipulation of the body achieved by rubbing, gently pinching, kneading, tapping, and performing other movements to increase metabolism and circulation, promote absorption, and relieve pain

_____ in massage, the rapid shaking movement in which the esthetician uses the body and shoulders, not just the fingertips, to create the movement

_____ kneading movement that stimulates the underlying tissues; performed by lifting, squeezing, and pressing the tissue with a light, firm pressure

_____ gentle rhythmic pressure on the lymphatic system to detoxify and remove waste materials from the body more quickly

_____ light continuous stroking movement applied with the fingers (digital) or the palms (palmar) in a slow, rhythmic manner

_____ movements consisting of short, quick tapping and slapping movements

DISCOVERIES AND ACCOMPLISHMENTS

In the space below, list 10 key concepts discussed in this chapter. Share your list with some of the other students in your class. Discuss your lists and decide which 5 concepts are the most important. You may want to revise your list based on good ideas shared by your peers.

Discoveries:

_____

_____

_____

_____

_____

_____

_____

_____

_____

_____

_____

_____

List at least three things you have accomplished since your last entry that relate to your career goals and/or facial massage.

Accomplishments:

_____

_____

_____

_____

_____

_____

_____

_____

_____

_____

_____

EXAM REVIEW

MULTIPLE CHOICE

1. Why is facial massage not advised for a client undergoing cancer therapy?

    a. Massage increases lymph movement.

    b. Overstimulation of the skin interferes with drugs.

    c. Ingredients in products used neutralize some drugs.

    d. The light used counteracts chemotherapy.

2. Jesse is practicing facial massage on a classmate and reviewing his techniques by talking about what he is doing and why. Jesse says, "One area I am going to avoid tapping is your _____".

    a. forehead

    b. cheeks

    c. neck

    d. jawbone

3. A classmate asks you for the definition of *feathering*. You tell them it is the _____.

    a. use of feathers for soft touching during a massage

    b. use of quick, bird-like movements during a massage

    c. term for the slowing-down movements at the end of a massage

    d. practice of resting a client on a feather pillow during a massage

4. Massaging muscles with outward strokes prevents what?

    a. too much pressure on the muscles

    b. the client from randomly moving

    c. the release of cortisol

    d. skin damage that can cause wrinkling

5. How many teaspoons of product should you use on the facial area?

    a. 1

    b. 3

    c. 5

    d. 7

6. Jessica has sensitive skin, so you will not use which movements during her facial massage?

    a. any movement with pressure more than a light touch

    b. neither friction nor tapotement

    c. upward strokes

    d. neither effleurage nor scissoring

7. A relaxing massage depends on consistent repetitive movements. Before moving to the next movement, how many times do you typically repeat a movement?

    a. one to two times

    b. repeat movements for one minute

    c. once on each side

    d. three to six times

8. Because facial massage increases circulation, what is the result?

    a. Muscles in the face become weaker.

    b. The skin is oxygenated and receives more nutrients.

    c. The epidermis receives more carbon dioxide.

    d. There can be an increase in facial hair growth.

9. Facial massage contracts muscles and is relaxing. What structures are stimulated by massage?

    a. the sensory receptors on the face

    b. the muscle attachments to the underlying bones

    c. both muscle and nerve points

    d. the superficial facial muscles

10. After her facial massage, Naomi tells you see feels less stressed. Why does facial massage reduce stress?

    a. Serotonin levels have been reduced.

    b. Cortisol levels have been reduced.

    c. Serotonin levels have been increased.

    d. Cortisol levels have been increased.

11. In which direction should massage movements be on the side of the neck?

    a. upward because carotid blood flow is upward

    b. upward because jugular blood flow is upward

    c. downward because carotid blood flow is downward

    d. downward because jugular vein blood flow is downward

12. You are performing pétrissage on Claire's cheeks. What action should precede this movement?

    a. lift and pinch the fleshy part of her cheek

    b. turn her chin to the opposite side you are working on

    c. tap the forehead gently and move to the cheek

    d. tap on the zygomatic bone

13. Describe the movement you will use on Jenny's forehead at the end of her facial massage.

    a. Thumbs will be placed above eyebrows with varying pressure.

    b. Movement will vary in pressure, with the pressure slightly increasing.

    c. Movement will move scissor-like and slow.

    d. Movement will become slower and slower, and touch will become lighter and lighter

14. What technique is used for lymph drainage?

    a. aggressive, irregular pressure

    b. gentle rhythmic pressure

    c. deep inward pressure at each point

    d. hard kneading movements

15. What term is used to describe manual movements used to increase metabolism and circulation?

    a. massage

    b. acupuncture

    c. physical therapy

    d. reconditioning

16. Which of the following improves overall metabolism and activates sluggish skin?

    a. caffeine

    b. massage therapy

    c. sun exposure

    d. diet high in protein

17. What should be performed for approximately 10 to 20 minutes during a facial?

    a. extractions

    b. facial massage

    c. steaming

    d. manicure

18. What qualification must estheticians have be in order to perform deep tissue work?

   a. licensed massage therapist (LMT)

   b. emergency medical technician (EMT)

   c. licensed medical technician (LMT)

   d. emergency massage technician (EMT)

19. Where should massage movements begin?

   a. insertion

   b. origin

   c. joint

   d. any point along the muscle

20. Clients sometimes have inflamed acne, open lesions, or sunburn. What massage is recommended for these conditions?

   a. Clients with these conditions need therapeutic massage.

   b. Massage is contraindicated for clients with these conditions.

   c. Clients with these conditions should receive only gentle massage.

   d. Clients with these conditions should receive only vigorous massage.

21. When should you avoid vigorous massage?

   a. when you are too tired to perform vigorous massage

   b. when clients have diabetes

   c. when a client has sensitive or redness-prone skin

   d. when a client has oily skin

22. One of your friends wants to try a facial massage, but she has reservations because of several health concerns. When should she consult her physician?

   a. after the first massage session

   b. before having a massage

   c. after a month of regular massage

   d. after a year of regular massage

23. You are gloved and ready to apply product for a facial massage. You take the container and remove the appropriate amount. Where should you place the product?

   a. in even amounts on your gloved hand

   b. on the neck of your client

   c. on a disposable cotton pad

   d. evenly dispersed on the client's right and left cheek

24. Alexis is dealing with a lot of stress and thinks a facial massage will help her. Which of the following could you add to her treatment to help her relax mentally?

    a. cold towels

    b. abrasion

    c. waxing

    d. essential oils

25. What types of movements are used in pétrissage?

    a. kneading

    b. hacking

    c. vibration

    d. tapping

26. Clients report feeling happier after a facial massage. What chemicals may be released during massage that promote feelings of well-being?

    a. dopamine and serotonin

    b. cortisol and dopamine

    c. cortisol and serotonin

    d. dopamine and epinephrine

27. Which of the following is NOT a benefit of facial massage?

    a. relieves muscle pain

    b. improves metabolism

    c. helps with product absorption

    d. reduces cancer risk

28. During a facial massage, why must the pressure be light on the side of the face?

    a. to avoid dragging the skin downward

    b. to vary the pressure, which relaxes the client

    c. because the temple region is sensitive to touch

    d. to avoid any dental issues the client may have

29. Estheticians must maintain hand mobility with specific exercises to reduce the risk of which occupational problem?

    a. shoulder pain

    b. carpal tunnel syndrome

    c. osteoarthritis

    d. tennis elbow (tendonitis)

30. When do the body's reflex receptors increase blood and lymph flow, resulting in a state of relaxation?
    a. when touch is sensed by the body
    b. when heat is sensed by the body
    c. when cold is sensed by the body
    d. when moisture is sensed by the body

31. What does the central nervous system trigger when massage is performed?
    a. rapid heartbeat
    b. "fight-or-flight" reaction
    c. stress
    d. relaxation

32. To whom should you refer a client who wants a therapeutic massage?
    a. physical therapist
    b. nurse practitioner
    c. licensed massage therapist
    d. chiropractor

33. What information can be found by referring to licensing regulations?
    a. product ingredients
    b. pricing scales
    c. scope of practice
    d. customer demographics

34. During a facial massage, a client suddenly jerks back and says that she was scratched. Which technique should be avoided to prevent this?
    a. avoid using lotions that might make the work surface slippery
    b. avoid using the ends of your fingertips
    c. avoid working in a warmth that might induce client perspiration
    d. avoid thick gloves to ensure they don't scratch the client's skin

35. What directions should the hands move around the eye and zygomatic region during facial massage?
    a. Left hand is clockwise; right hand is counter-clockwise.
    b. Left hand is counter-clockwise; right hand is clockwise.
    c. Both hands move clockwise in synchrony.
    d. Both hands move counter-clockwise in synchrony.

36. In order to not damage tissue, how long should vibration last on any one spot of the body?

    a. no more than a few seconds

    b. no more than a minute

    c. no more than 10 minutes

    d. no more than 20 minutes

37. What should an esthetician understand about massaging both sides of the face?

    a. The left side should receive more vigorous massage.

    b. The right side should receive more vigorous massage.

    c. Use the right hand on the left side and the left hand on the right side.

    d. Movements should be duplicated on both the right and left sides.

38. After a facial massage, your client comments that part of the massage felt like you were playing a piano! You tell him there is a name for that technique. It is called _____.

    a. tapotement

    b. vibration

    c. effleurage

    d. feathering

39. Patients with what contraindication(s) can now receive facial massage without concern, especially if the condition is being treated by a physician?

    a. inflamed acne

    b. skin disorders

    c. diabetes

    d. sunburn

40. Devan comes in regularly for a facial massage and you are comfortable with the procedure you typically use. When you greet him, you see that he now has a beard. What type of movements are you going to use because of the beard?

    a. downward

    b. upward

    c. sideways

    d. diagonal

PROCEDURE 9–1: PERFORM A BASIC FACIAL MASSAGE

Evaluate your practical skills.

CRITERIA	COMPETENT	NEEDS WORK	IMPROVEMENT PLAN
Preparation			
Perform Procedure 7–1: Pre-Service—Preparing the Treatment Room.			
Perform Procedure 8–1: Pre-Service—Preparing the Client for Treatment.			
Application of Facial Massage Product			
1. Dispense the massage product. Safely dispense the correct product for the client's skin type and needs into a container. One teaspoon (5 millimeters or 5 to 10 grams) should be enough product for the facial area, neck, and décolleté.			
2. Put on gloves and prepare massage product. Put on well-fitting gloves to perform the facial massage properly. Ensure the massage cream is evenly distributed on both gloved hands. You are now ready to apply the product to the client's décolleté (includes the upper chest area, neck, and cleavage) and face.			
3. Use effleurage to apply product evenly to the décolleté, neck, and face. While applying the product, it is suggested that hands not be lifted from the client until you are finished. Start applying a small amount of the product by placing both hands, palms down, on the décolleté. Slide hands across the décolleté toward the shoulders, back to the center of the décolleté, up the neck to the face, out to the cheeks; then glide inward, up the nose, and end the application by tapering the movement off until the fingers are gradually lifted from the forehead, a process also referred to as feathering.			
Facial Massage Routine			
Optional: Begin massage with décolleté, shoulder, and neck manipulations as discussed on page 408 and then proceed to step 1 below or perform only the massage steps as listed below.			
1. Start with hands on the décolleté. Using your full hands, including the palms, move slowly up the sides of the neck and face to the forehead. Beginning on the forehead, slide to each of the next steps without breaking contact or lifting fingers off the face.			

2. Effleurage strokes on the forehead. With the middle and ring fingers of each hand, start upward strokes in the middle of the forehead, starting at the brow line and moving upward toward the hairline. Move toward the right temple and back to the center of the forehead. Now move toward the left temple and back to the center of the forehead. Repeat three to six times.			
3. Circular friction on the forehead. With the middle or index finger of each hand, start a circular movement in the middle of the forehead along the brow line. Continue this circular movement while working toward the temples. Each time the fingers reach the temples, pause for a moment and apply slight pressure to the temples. Make sure the pressure is acceptable to your client. Bring the fingers back to the center of the forehead at a point between the brow line and the hairline. Move up on the forehead toward the hairline for the final movements. Repeat three to six times.			
4. Friction using crisscross strokes on the forehead. With the middle and ring fingers of each hand, start a criss-cross stroking movement at the middle of the forehead, starting at the brow line and moving upward toward the hairline. Move toward the right temple and back to the center of the forehead. Now move toward the left temple and back to the center of the forehead. Repeat three to six times.			
5. Friction near the brows. Place the ring fingers under the inside corners of the eyebrows and the middle fingers over the brows. Slide the fingers to the outer corner of each eye, lifting the brow at the same time. This movement continues with the next step.			
6. Circular friction around the eye area and zygomatic. Start a circular movement with the middle and ring fingers at the inside corner of each eye. Continue the circular movement on the zygomatic bone (cheekbone) to the point under the center of the eye, and then slide the fingers back to the starting point. Repeat three to six times. The left hand moves clockwise, and the right hand moves counter-clockwise.			
7. Tapotement around the eyes. Start a light tapping movement with the pads of the fingers. Tap lightly around the eyes as if gently playing a piano. Continue tapping, moving from the temple to under the eye, toward the nose, up and over the brow, and outward back to the temple. Do not tap the eyelids directly over the eyeball. Repeat the movements three to six times.			
8. Circular friction across the cheeks to the temples and back. With the middle, index, or ring finger of each hand, start a circular movement down the nose and continue across the cheeks to the temples. Slide the fingers under the eyes and back to the bridge of the nose. Repeat the movements three to six times.			

9. Pétrissage motion on the chin. With the middle and ring fingers of each hand, slide the fingers from the bridge of the nose, over the brow (lifting the brow), and down to the chin. Start a firm circular movement on the chin with the thumbs. Change to the middle fingers at the corners of the mouth. Rotate the fingers five times, and slide the fingers up the sides of the nose and over the brow, and then stop for a moment at the temples. Apply slight pressure on the temples. Slide the fingers down to the chin, and repeat the movements three to six times. The downward movement on the side of the face should have a very light touch to avoid dragging the skin downward.			
10. Perform tapotement or pétrissage on the cheeks. a. If using pétrissage, grasp the skin between the thumb and forefinger of the index finger, gently lift and pinch the fleshy areas of the cheeks with light but firm pressure. Remember to use this type of pétrissage movement only on the fleshy areas of the face. Work in a circle around the cheeks. Repeat the movements three to six times. b. If using tapotement, start a light tapping motion (piano playing) on the cheeks, working in a circle around the cheeks. Repeat three to six times.			
11. Circular friction or rubbing motion. Slide to the center of the chin. Using the middle and ring fingers of each hand, start a circular movement at the center of the chin and move up to the earlobes. Slide the middle fingers to the corners of the mouth and then continue the circular movements to the middle of the ears. Return the middle fingers to the nose and continue the circular movements outward across the cheeks to the top of the ear. Repeat each of the three passes three to six times. Slide down to the mouth.			
12. Friction using scissoring movement. Place the index finger above the mouth and middle finger below the mouth. Start the "scissor" movement, gliding from the center of the mouth and upward over the zygomatic bone (cheekbone), and stopping at the top of the zygomatic. Alternate the movement from one side of the face to the other, using the right hand on the right side of the face and then the left hand on the left side. As one hand reaches the zygomatic bone (cheekbone), start the other at the center of the mouth. Repeat the movements three to six times.			
13. Circle around the mouth and chin. With the middle fingers of both hands, draw the fingers from the center of the upper lip around the mouth and under the lower lip, and then continue a circle under the chin. Repeat the movements three to six times.			

14. Friction using scissor movement. With the index finger above the chin and jawline (the middle, ring, and little fingers should be under the chin and jaw), start a scissor movement from the center of the chin and then slide the fingers along the jawline to the earlobe. Alternate one hand after the other, using the right hand on the right side of the face and the left hand on the left side of the face. Repeat three to six times on each side of the face. Slide down to the neck.			
15. Effleurage near the neck. Using both hands, apply light upward strokes over the front of the neck. Circle down and then back up, using firmer downward pressure on the outer sides of the neck. Repeat the movements three to six times. Do not press down on the center of the neck.			
16. Tapotement on the underside of the chin. With the middle and ring fingers of the right hand, give two quick taps under the chin, followed with one quick tap with the middle and ring fingers of the left hand. The taps should be done in a continuous movement, keeping a steady rhythm. The taps should be done with a light touch, but with enough pressure so that a soft tapping sound can be heard. Continue the tapping movement while moving the hands slightly to the right and then to the left, so as to cover the complete underside of the chin. Without stopping or breaking the rhythm of the tapping, move to the right cheek.			
17. Tapotement and lifting movement on the cheeks. Continue the tapping on the right cheek in the same manner as under the chin, except the tapping with the left hand will have a lifting movement. The rhythm will be tap, tap, lift, tap, tap, lift, tap, tap, lift. Repeat this rhythmic movement three to six times. Without stopping the tapping movement, move the fingers back under the chin and over the left cheek, repeating the tapping and lifting movements. Move up and out of the area in a consistent pattern. Avoid tapping directly on the jawbone because this will feel unpleasant to the client.			
18. Tapotement stroking movement near corners of the mouth. Without stopping the tapping movement, move the hands over to the corners of the mouth. Break into an upward stroking movement with the first three fingers of each hand. One finger follows the other as each finger lifts the corner of the mouth. Use both hands at the same time or alternate each hand—as one hand ends the movement, the other starts. Repeat the stroking movement three to six times.			

19. Effleurage stroking movement near outside corner of eyes. Without stopping the stroking movement, move up to the outside corner of the left eye and continue the stroking upward movement. Continue the stroking movement across the forehead to the outside corner of the right eye. Continue this stroking movement back and forth three to six times in each direction.			
20. Effleurage stroking movement across the forehead and complete routine. Continue the stroking movement back and forth across the forehead, gradually slowing the movement. Let the movements grow slower and slower as the touch becomes lighter and lighter. Taper the movement off until the fingers are gradually lifted from the forehead.			
21. Remove the massage medium. Use warm towels or 4" × 4" esthetics wipes and follow the same procedure for removing other products or cleansers. Continue with the facial service.			
Post-Service			
Complete Procedure 7–2: Post-Service Procedure.			

CHAPTER 10
FACIAL DEVICES AND TECHNOLOGY

EXPLAIN THE IMPORTANCE OF THE USE OF FACIAL DEVICES AND TECHNOLOGY

SHORT ESSAY

1. Tracy is studying to become an esthetician. Give three reasons why she needs to have a thorough understanding of facial machines.

_____

_____

_____

_____

_____

_____

_____

_____

_____

_____

_____

_____

_____

IDENTIFY THE BASIC CONCEPTS OF ELECTROTHERAPY

FILL IN THE BLANK

2. Electrical devices enhance facial treatments by _____, by _____, or by _____.

3. These tools are especially effective for more challenging skin conditions such as
_____.

4. It is important to be familiar with machines and devices even if you choose not to work with them, as it is important to be able to _____.

General Contraindications for Electrotherapy

SHORT ANSWER

5. List five characteristics of clients who should NOT receive electrotherapy.

    1. _____

    2. _____

    3. _____

    4. _____

    5. _____

EXPLAIN THE BENEFITS OF THE HOT TOWEL CABINET

SHORT ANSWER

6. Why would you use a hot towel cabinet?

_____

_____

When to Use a Hot Towel Cabinet

FILL IN THE BLANK

7. Hot towels can be used for _____ treatments.

8. UV lamps in towel warmers may _____ but are not effective for _____.

Effects of Warm Towels from a Hot Towel Cabinet

SHORT ANSWER

9. What are the effects of using warm towels?

    • _____

    • _____

    • _____

Contraindications and Best Practices for Warm Towels from a Hot Towel Cabinet

SHORT ANSWER

10. List three contraindications for warm towels from a hot towel cabinet.

- _____

- _____

- _____

11. List three best practices for preparing hot towels.

- _____
  _____

- _____
  _____

- _____
  _____

12. What steps should be followed to prepare the hot towel cabinet?

1. _____
   _____

2. _____
   _____

3. _____
   _____

Safety and Maintenance of the Hot Towel Cabinet

CASE STUDY

13. **Towel Treatment**

    Faith is about to use a heated steam towel from her hot towel cabinet. What steps should she take when applying the towel to her waiting client?

    _____

    _____

    _____

    _____

    _____

    _____

14. **Cabinet Cleanup**

   Faith just said goodbye to her last client of the day and is about to clean the hot towel cabinet. What steps should she take to clean the towel cabinet?

   _____

   _____

   _____

   _____

   _____

   _____

DISCUSS THE MAGNIFYING LAMP AND ITS USES

SHORT ANSWER

15. Describe how a magnifying lamp works.

   _____

   _____

   _____

   _____

   _____

   _____

When to Use the Magnifying Lamp

SHORT ANSWER

16. When would you use a magnifying lamp during client treatments?

   • _____

   • _____

   • _____

Best Practices for the Magnifying Lamp

FILL IN THE BLANK

17. _____ are not as mobile, so _____ are preferred for the base of a magnifying lamp.

18. Always use _____ when using a magnifying lamp directly over the client.

19. Avoid adjusting a lamp's _____ over the client's face or body.

Safety and Maintenance of the Magnifying Lamp

SHORT ANSWER

20. What is the correct way to clean the lens of a magnifying lamp?

_____

_____

_____

_____

_____

DISCUSS THE WOOD'S LAMP AND ITS USES

FILL IN THE BLANK

21. A Wood's lamp uses a filtered _____ light to illuminate _____, _____ disorders, _____ problems, and other _____ problems.

22. _____ are similar to Wood's lamps. These larger _____ analysis tools use a _____ light with an interior _____.

When to Use the Wood's Lamp

SHORT ANSWER

23. Complete the **Wood's Lamp Reference Chart** for various skin conditions.

Skin Condition	Appearance Under Wood's Lamp
Thick corneum layer	
Horny layer of dead skin cells	
Normal, healthy skin	
Thin or dehydrated skin	
Acne or bacteria	
Oily areas of the face/comedones	
Hyperpigmentation or sun damage	
Hypopigmentation	

FILL IN THE BLANK

24. What pigmentation can be potentially lightened by exfoliation treatments and lightening products?

_____

Contraindications and Best Practices for the Wood's Lamp & Safety and Maintenance of the Wood's Lamp

TRUE OR FALSE

25. For the following statements on using and storing the Wood's lamp, circle *T* if true or *F* if false.

T   F   When using the Wood's lamp, the room must be totally dark.

T   F   Place small eye pads on the client, making sure the area around the eye is completely covered.

T   F   The bulbs used do not get hot, so pose no danger to skin.

T   F   A large open plastic tub is helpful for storing all of the glass parts of various tools and machines.

DEMONSTRATE HOW TO SAFELY AND EFFECTIVELY USE THE ROTARY BRUSH

FILL IN THE BLANK

26. The main purpose of the rotary brush is to _____ the skin.

27. Brushes come in smaller sizes for _____ and larger sizes for _____, with different _____ ranging from soft to firm.

When to Use the Rotary Brush & Effects of the Rotary Brush

TRUE OR FALSE

28. For the following statements on use of the rotary brush, circle *T* if true or *F* if false.

T   F   Use the brush when your goal is to lightly exfoliate the skin with the use of chemicals such as enzymes or peels.

T   F   Using the rotary brush during the second cleansing step in a facial saves time for both you and your client.

T   F   Cleansing brushes can soothe the skin and help stimulate oil secretion.

Contraindications and Best Practices for the Rotary Brush

SHORT ANSWER

29. List four contraindications for the rotary brush.

- _____
- _____
- _____
- _____

30. List three best practices for the rotary brush.

- _____

- _____

- _____

Safety and Maintenance of the Rotary Brush

SHORT ANSWER

31. Describe how to disinfect and maintain rotary brushes.

1. _____

2. _____

3. _____

4. _____

5. When the brushes are completely dry, transfer them to a closed container.

DEMONSTRATE HOW TO SAFELY AND EFFECTIVELY USE THE STEAMER

TRUE OR FALSE

32. For the following statements on the steamer, circle *T* if true or *F* if false.

T F   Use only distilled water in a steamer.

T F   The steamer takes approximately four to five minutes to heat up.

T F   Do not direct the arm of the steamer toward the client's face.

T F   Essential oils should be added directly to the steamer's water reservoir to promote proper diffusion.

When to Use the Steamer

FILL IN THE BLANK

33. The steamer is typically used during the _____ in a facial.

34. It can be used prior to _____ to _____ the skin.

35. It can be used to soften a _____ and facilitate its _____.

Effects of the Steamer

SHORT ANSWER

36. List three benefits of using the steamer during a service.

- _____

  _____

- _____

  _____

- _____

  _____

Contraindications and Best Practices for the Steamer

FILL IN THE BLANK

37. Complete the following contraindications and best practices for the steamer.

- Do not use too much steam on _____, because it can cause more redness and irritation.

- Avoid placing the steamer arm _____.

- Never touch _____ on the steamer when it is hot.

- Do not _____ while steaming the client in case the steamer starts spraying water.

- Do not _____ the steamer because it may spray excess water and burn the client.

- Clean the steamer regularly to _____ that causes water to spray.

- Do not _____ to the steamer until it has cooled off.

Safety and Maintenance of the Steamer

SHORT ANSWER

38. What should you do at night to maintain your steamer?

_____

_____

_____

_____

_____

39. What should you do each morning to maintain your steamer?

_____

_____

_____

_____

_____

40. Where do essential oils or herbs go in a steamer?

_____

_____

_____

_____

_____

41. What does an automatic regulator on a steamer do?

_____

_____

_____

_____

_____

PROCEDURE 10–1: USE OF AND CARE FOR THE STEAMER

FILL IN THE BLANK

42. Complete the steps of **Procedure 10–1A: Use the Steamer**.

   1. Perform Procedure 7–1: Pre-service—Preparing the Treatment Room.

   2. Place _____ into the designated container through the fill opening in the top. Check that it is _____ and is level with the _____ line.

   3. Perform an equipment precheck and _____ of your equipment. Do not position the steamer arm/nozzle _____. Wait until the steamer has _____ prior to directing on the client.

   4.–8. Prep and cleanse the client.

   9. Apply _____ or _____.

10. Turn on the steamer. If the steamer has a secondary option of
_____ or vapor, do not turn on the second switch until
_____.

11. When the water is boiling, and _____, slowly adjust the
steamer arm _____.

12. Keep the steam approximately _____ inches
(_____ centimeters) from the face.

13. Reposition the steamer as needed to get _____ across the
face.

14. Never _____ while steaming. Do not
_____ the skin. Steaming should last
_____ minutes.

15. When you are ready to discontinue the steam, _____ then
turn off the steamer.

16. Continue with the next step in the facial or close out this procedure.

17. Remove _____; apply
_____ and _____
protection.

18. Perform Procedure 8–9: Post-Service Procedure.

19. Perform Procedure 7–2: Post-Service—Clean-Up and Preparation for the Next Client.

DEMONSTRATE HOW TO SAFELY AND EFFECTIVELY USE THE VACUUM MACHINE

SHORT ANSWER

43. What are the uses of the vacuum machine?

_____

_____

_____

_____

_____

When to Use the Vacuum Machine & Effects of the Vacuum Machine

FILL IN THE BLANK

44. The vacuum machine can be used after _____ and before
_____ .

45. The vacuum machine can also be used in place of _____.

46. The vacuum machine is used to suction _____ from the skin, and to _____ the _____ layer as well as _____ and blood circulation.

Contraindications and Best Practices for the Vacuum Machine & Safety and Maintenance for the Vacuum Machine

SHORT ANSWER

47. Which three skin conditions should NOT receive vacuum machine treatment?

- _____
- _____
- _____

48. How can you avoid damaging the skin while using the vacuum machine?

_____
_____
_____
_____
_____

49. Where is the filter in a vacuum machine and how often should it be changed?

_____
_____
_____
_____
_____

DEMONSTRATE HOW TO SAFELY AND EFFECTIVELY USE GALVANIC CURRENT

SHORT ANSWER

50. Galvanic current is used to create two significant reactions in esthetics: _____
_____.

51. What is the result of electrons allowed to flow continuously in the same direction through a client?

_____
_____

When to Use Galvanic Current

FILL IN THE BLANK

52. Galvanic current can be used in a facial after the _____ step and prior to the
_____ step.

53. Galvanic current can be used prior to masking to _____ or during the final
stages of _____.

Effects of Using the Galvanic Machine

SHORT ANSWER / FILL IN THE BLANK

54. What does desincrustation do? _____

_____

_____

_____

_____

55. What does iontophoresis do? _____

_____

_____

_____

_____

56. What is saponification? _____

_____

_____

_____

_____

57. Why is the polarity of solutions important? _____

_____

_____

_____

_____

58. Mark the following effects with an *A* if they are caused by anaphoresis, or a *C* if they are caused by cataphoresis.

_____   increases blood circulation

_____   calms or soothes nerve endings

_____   softens and relaxes tissue

_____   causes an alkaline reaction

_____   decreases blood circulation

_____   causes an acidic reaction

_____   stimulates nerve endings

_____   tightens the skin

Contraindications and Best Practices for the Galvanic Machine & Safety and Maintenance of the Galvanic Machine

SHORT ANSWER

59. What are five contraindications for galvanic current?

_____

_____

_____

_____

_____

_____

60. What is the first step in cleaning and disinfecting galvanic electrodes?

_____

_____

_____

_____

_____

61. How long should you sterilize a metal electrode in an autoclave?

_____

_____

_____

_____

_____

PROCEDURE 10-2: PERFORM DESINCRUSTATION AND IONTOPHORESIS USING THE GALVANIC MACHINE

FILL IN THE BLANK

62. Place the following steps of Part 1: Desincrustation in the correct order. Start with 1 and end with 8.

_____ Apply the electrode to the client's forehead. Make sure the electrode is directly on the skin before turning on the galvanic current.

_____ Cover the entire positive electrode that makes contact with the client with a piece of dampened cotton around the electrode. Give this to the client to hold or place behind the client's shoulder.

_____ Continue in the T-zone area down the nose and into the chin area (or into any area that is oily or needs desincrustation). Avoid areas with dry skin conditions.

_____ Gently rotate the electrode while gliding it over the client's face. Do not lift the electrode or break contact once the machine is on the skin, or it will be uncomfortable for the client. Keep the electrode as flat as possible and parallel to the skin's surface at all times.

_____ Keep the electrode constantly moving to avoid overstimulating an area. Keep the skin moist. Add water to face if it gets too dry to glide over the skin.

_____ Apply desincrustation fluid to the entire face and then apply the precut gauze face mask over the face.

_____ Turn the switch to negative and set at the appropriate level for the client.

_____ When you are finished, turn off the machine first and then remove the electrode. Rinse the skin thoroughly with moistened esthetic wipes.

63. Place the following steps of Part 2: Iontophoresis in the correct order. Start with 1 and end with 8.

_____ Cover the entire positive electrode that makes contact with the client with a piece of dampened cotton around the electrode. Give this to the client to hold or place behind the client's shoulder.

_____ You have the option of switching positive and negative poles when infusing solutions. Consult the product manufacturer's instructions when doing so.

_____ When you are finished, turn off the machine first and then remove the electrode. Remove the gauze and rinse the skin thoroughly.

_____ Beginning on the forehead, gently rotate the electrode while gliding it over the client's forehead. Do not lift the electrode or break contact once the machine is on the skin, or it will be uncomfortable for the client. Keep the electrode as flat as possible and parallel to the skin's surface at all times.

_____ Continue to the cheeks and the rest of the face.

_____ Apply ampoule or serum to the entire face and then apply the precut gauze face mask over the face.

_____ Dip the electrode into water or a conductive gel solution. Apply the electrode to the client's forehead. Make sure the electrode is directly on the skin before turning on the galvanic current.

_____ Keep the electrode constantly moving to avoid overstimulating an area. Keep the skin moist and the pads wet. Add water to the pad or face if it gets too dry to glide over the skin.

DEMONSTRATE HOW TO SAFELY AND EFFECTIVELY USE THE HIGH-FREQUENCY MACHINE

FILL IN THE BLANK

64. The high-frequency machine utilizes an _____ or sinusoidal current and produces _____.

65. High-frequency current basically has _____ polarity and in effect does not produce _____. This makes _____ physically impossible.

Electrodes

FILL IN THE BLANK

66. Mark the following characteristics with an *N* if they relate to electrodes of neon gas, or an *A* if they relate to those of argon.

_____ red

_____ for acne-prone skin

_____ violet

_____ for aging skin

_____ blue

_____ orange

_____ for normal to oily skin

_____ pink

_____ for sensitive skin

67. Complete the **High-Frequency Electrode Reference Table**.

Electrode	General Application
_____ (small or large)	• _____ the electrode over _____ in _____ movements (across the forehead) and then to the nose, cheeks, and chin area. • Can be used to produce a _____ onto the skin; ideal for _____ or _____ skin. • High frequency may be used at the end of a _____ treatment over _____.
_____ (spiral)	• Used to _____ during massage. This treatment is ideal for _____ and _____ skin.
_____ (glass tip)	• Used to _____ to a specific area such as _____, helping to _____.
_____ (rake)	• Used mainly in a _____ treatment.

When to Use High Frequency & Effects of High Frequency

SHORT ANSWER

68. When can high frequency be applied?

_____

_____

_____

_____

_____

69. What are three benefits the high-frequency machine can have on skin?

- _____

   _____

   _____

   _____

- _____

   _____

   _____

   _____

- _____

   _____

   _____

   _____

Contraindications and Best Practices for High Frequency

FILL IN THE BLANK

70. To avoid being burned, avoid _____ during electrical machine treatments.

71. Clients should _____ prior to the treatment.

72. The esthetician should _____ on the electrode prior to applying it to the client and prior to removing if from _____.

73. The electrode should be _____ at all times.

Safety and Maintenance for High Frequency

TRUE OR FALSE

74. For the following statements on high-frequency machine maintenance, circle *T* if true or *F* if false.

T   F   Clean the electrode by wiping it with a solution of soap and water.

T   F   Use alcohol on electrodes if available.

T   F   Always submerge electrodes completely in water.

T   F   Dry electrodes with a clean towel and store in an airtight closed container.

T   F   Use an autoclave to sterilize electrodes for added safety.

T   F   Replace electrodes regularly.

T   F   Cover electrodes so they remain clean and undamaged.

T   F   The high-frequency coil built into the machine does not require replacing.

T   F   Clean the hand piece, cords, and machine with disinfectant.

DEMONSTRATE HOW TO SAFELY AND EFFECTIVELY USE THE SPRAY MACHINE

FILL IN THE BLANK

75. Spray mists are beneficial in _____ and _____ the skin.

76. The spray machine is part of the _____ machine.

When to Use a Spray Machine & Effects of Using the Spray Machine

SHORT ANSWER

77. When would you use a spray machine?

_____

_____

_____

78. What is the benefit of using the spray machine?

_____

_____

_____

Contraindications and Best Practices for the Spray Machine & Safety and Maintenance for the Spray Machine

SHORT ANSWER

79. List the guidelines for safely using the spray machine.

- _____
  _____

- _____
  _____

- _____
  _____

- _____
  _____

- _____
  _____

- _____
  _____

STATE THE BENEFITS AND USE OF PARAFFIN WAX

SHORT ANSWER

80. What are two modern methods of paraffin wax application that prevent cross-contamination?

_____
_____
_____
_____
_____

When to Use Paraffin Wax & Effects of Using Paraffin Wax

FILL IN THE BLANK

81. The warm paraffin mask is used for _____ and is generally applied over a _____ to the hands and feet.

82. Paraffin wax allows the esthetician to provide a treatment that _____, but it _____.

Contraindications and Best Practices of Paraffin Wax & Safety and Maintenance

TRUE OR FALSE

83. For the following statements on the use of paraffin wax, circle *T* if true or *F* if false.

    T   F   Wax treatments are safe for all skin types and conditions, due to the mild temperatures involved.

    T   F   Paraffin wax heaters stay warm at a safe, low level of heat.

    T   F   These heaters heat up quickly but should still be switched on at the very beginning of a service.

    T   F   A substitute heater, such as an electric cooking pot, is also recommended in case the wax heater fails.

    T   F   The use of separate heaters for applications for the hands and the feet prevents cross-contamination.

STATE THE BENEFITS AND USE OF THE ELECTRIC MITTS AND BOOTS

FILL IN THE BLANK

84. Electric boots and mitts are similar to _____ and have

_____.

When to Use Electric Mitts and Boots & Effects of Electric Mitts and Boots

SHORT ANSWER

85. List the uses of electric mitts and boots.

    • _____

    _____

    • _____

    _____

Contraindications and Best Practices of Electric Mitts and Boots & Safety and Maintenance of the Electric Mitts and Boots

SHORT ANSWER

86. Why should you avoid allowing the warmers to get too hot?

_____

_____

_____

_____

_____

87. How should you clean electric mitts and boots?

_____

_____

_____

_____

_____

IDENTIFY WHY YOU SHOULD MAKE AN INFORMED DECISION WHEN PURCHASING EQUIPMENT AS A LICENSED ESTHETICIAN

SHORT ANSWER

88. What information should you gather about any new equipment before purchasing?

- _____
- _____
- _____
- _____
- _____

WORD REVIEW

MATCHING

89. Match the term to its definition.

a. ions	d. Wood's lamp	g. rotary brush
b. saponification	e. high-frequency machine	h. sinusoidal current
c. thermolysis	f. vacuum machine	i. spray machine

_____ apparatus that utilizes alternating current to produce a mild to strong heat effect

_____ also known as *suction machine*

_____ machine used to lightly exfoliate and stimulate the skin; also helps soften excess oil, dirt, and cell buildup

_____ chemical reaction during desincrustation where the current transforms the sebum into soap

_____ heat effect; used for permanent hair removal

_____ atoms or molecules that carry an electrical charge

_____ a smooth, repetitive alternating current

_____ spray misting device

_____ filtered black light that is used to illuminate skin disorders, fungi, bacterial disorders, and pigmentation

DISCOVERIES AND ACCOMPLISHMENTS

In the space below, write five notes about key concepts discussed in this chapter. Share your discoveries with other students in your class and ask them if your notes are helpful to them. Then write five more notes based on discoveries that your peers shared with you.

Discoveries:

_____

_____

_____

_____

_____

_____

_____

_____

_____

_____

_____

List at least three things you have accomplished since your last entry that relate to your career goals.

Accomplishments:

_____

_____

_____

_____

_____

_____

_____

_____

_____

_____

_____

EXAM REVIEW

MULTIPLE CHOICE

1. How does dehydrated skin appear under a Wood's lamp?

    a. light violet/purple

    b. light turquoise/blue

    c. deep crimson/red

    d. deep emerald/green

2. Which of the following is needed to maintain professional credibility?

    a. understanding the contraindications in using machines and devices

    b. operating machines and devices safely

    c. the ability to explain the benefits of each machine and device

    d. continued education about the latest methods in skin care

3. Sasha has a client with hypopigmentation. She discovers this by looking at the client's skin under a Wood's lamp. How does the client's skin appear?

    a. red-purple or beige-brown

    b. blue-white or yellow-green

    c. orange-yellow or gray-black

    d. black-red or brown-gray

4. Mackenzie's client asks for help with excess cell buildup, excess dirt, and excess oil. Which tool will Mackenzie use on her client?

    a. steamer

    b. rotary brush

    c. galvanic current

    d. electric mitts

5. How can you prevent cross-contamination when using a paraffin wax heater?

    a. use a plastic sleeve

    b. use an electric cooking pot

    c. keep wax at a high heat level

    d. use new wax for each client

6. How often should you remove brushes from the rotary brush machine, wash them with soap and water, and immerse them in disinfectant per manufacturer recommendations?

    a. once per day

    b. once per week

    c. after every client

    d. after every few clients

7. Why should you avoid using tap water in steamers?

    a. Calcium buildups in tap water necessitate extra cleaning.

    b. Mineral deposits in tap water give steam an unpleasant odor.

    c. Calcium and mineral deposits in tap water might damage machinery.

    d. Tap water is not thick enough to be used with a steamer.

8. What function does the rotary brush perform?

    a. aggressive extraction

    b. gentle extraction

    c. light exfoliation

    d. heavy exfoliation

9. What is sebum transformed into via the chemical reaction of saponification?

    a. lymph

    b. soap

    c. oil

    d. cold cream

10. What is NOT true of sinusoidal current?

    a. It is a smooth, repetitive current.

    b. It is an alternating current.

    c. It produces heat effects.

    d. Use on the scalp is contraindicated.

11. What is a misting device used for facial treatments?

    a. spray machine

    b. vacuum machine

    c. high-frequency machine

    d. steamer

12. What is a heat effect that is used for permanent hair removal?

    a. saponification

    b. desincrustation

    c. anaphoresis

    d. thermolysis

13. What is the purpose of a vacuum machine?

    a. cleaning up debris after facial treatments

    b. removing impurities and stimulating circulation

    c. quickly removing makeup before a facial treatment

    d. extracting fine facial hairs left behind after shaving

14. What type of light does a Wood's lamp use?

    a. white light

    b. blue light

    c. red light

    d. black light

15. When should you ask a client to get a doctor's note?

    a. prior to any facial services

    b. prior to using facial machines

    c. if you have doubts about whether the client can have electrotherapy

    d. if you have doubts about whether the client practices good home care

16. Kimberly is about to begin using an electrical device on a client when she notices that the client is wearing jewelry. When should she have the client remove her jewelry?

    a. when she gets close to working in the area of the jewelry

    b. only if the jewelry is large and cumbersome

    c. before beginning the procedure

    d. after completing the procedure

17. Cassandra just ordered several new sets of mitts and boots for her spa. How should she clean them?

    a. spray with an essential oil and store in a dry container

    b. wipe with a disinfectant after each use

    c. flush with distilled water

    d. wipe with a solution of soap and water

18. What do electric mitts and boots do?
    a. increase cell metabolism
    b. help lotion penetrate
    c. hydrate dry skin
    d. calm the skin

19. What is emulsified or liquefied during desincrustation?
    a. sebum and debris
    b. lymph and debris
    c. oil and water
    d. lymph and water

20. What is the term for the use of electronic devices for therapeutic benefits?
    a. electrified therapy
    b. electrolysis
    c. electrotherapy
    d. electronic therapy

21. What is NOT true of galvanic current?
    a. It is a constant current.
    b. It is a direct current.
    c. It produces chemical reactions.
    d. It is contraindicated for the face.

22. What sort of effect is generated by a high-frequency machine?
    a. gentle warming
    b. strong heat
    c. gentle cooling
    d. strong cold

23. What are ions?
    a. atoms or molecules carrying a negative electrical charge
    b. atoms or molecules carrying a positive electrical charge
    c. atoms or molecules carrying an electrical charge
    d. atoms or molecules that cannot carry an electrical charge

24. What is ionization?
    a. process of fortifying a substance with additional ions
    b. process of separating a substance into ions
    c. process of identifying and cataloguing ions
    d. process of merging ions to form a new substance

25. Nichole is preparing her steamer and notices that steam is visible. What should she do?
    a. begin the treatment without any further steps
    b. turn on the second switch (the ozone or vaporizer)
    c. turn off the second switch (the ozone or vaporizer)
    d. turn the device off to prevent it from overheating

26. Many of Maggie's clients have requested that she use the steamer. What should Maggie do with her steamer after each use?
    a. turn it off for one hour
    b. clean and disinfect it
    c. top off the water in the reservoir
    d. add bleach to the water in the reservoir to prevent bacterial growth

27. What is NOT true about essential oils as they relate to the process of using a steamer?
    a. They should be placed in a wick-like apparatus near the nozzle.
    b. They should be deposited directly into the steamer's water supply.
    c. Essential oils require different equipment than herbs do.
    d. Essential oils can be a helpful addition to a steam treatment.

28. Rika is excited to use her new vacuum machine. She suggests it to a client to replace what treatment?
    a. product application
    b. steam treatment
    c. massage
    d. extractions

29. Erica is cautious to avoid lifting her finger off the hold of a vacuum machine in order to avoid causing what kind of discomfort to her clients?
    a. infecting the skin
    b. burning the skin
    c. cutting the skin
    d. pulling the skin

30. What sort of storage is appropriate for vacuum-machine tips?
    a. heated
    b. refrigerated
    c. covered
    d. uncovered

31. Talya recommends desincrustation to a client. What type of skin does the client have?
    a. normal
    b. mature
    c. dry
    d. oily

32. Where is an appropriate place to warm cotton pads and products?
    a. microwave
    b. hot plate
    c. paraffin wax heater
    d. towel warmer

33. How often should you clean the inside of the hot-towel cabinet with a topical disinfectant?
    a. once per day
    b. once per week
    c. once every hour
    d. after each client session

34. What should you do to the water catchment tray underneath the hot-towel cabinet's caddy on a daily basis?
    a. simply wipe it down with a paper towel
    b. rinse it with water and let it air dry
    c. empty, clean, and disinfect it
    d. discard and replace it

35. What is the most common magnification for magnifying lamps, measured in diopters?
    a. 5
    b. 10
    c. 15
    d. 20

36. What is NOT a common cause of eyestrain?

    a. steam in the treatment room

    b. improper illumination

    c. distortion on the magnifying lamp

    d. insufficient illumination

37. What is sometimes known as a "loupe"?

    a. tweezers

    b. Wood's lamp

    c. magnifying lamp

    d. steamer

38. When should you loosen the adjustment knobs on your magnifying lamp?

    a. at the start of every day

    b. at the end of every day

    c. never

    d. whenever you move the arms

39. What should you AVOID using on the lens of your magnifying lamp?

    a. lens tissue

    b. lens-cleaning fluid

    c. paper products

    d. soft cloth

40. Abigail is about to purchase new equipment for her spa. Which of the following is NOT a consideration for her?

    a. warranties and training

    b. insurance coverage

    c. cost to clients

    d. regulations

PROCEDURE 10–1: USE AND CARE FOR THE STEAMER

Evaluate your practical skills.

CRITERIA	COMPETENT	NEEDS WORK	IMPROVEMENT PLAN
A. Use the Steamer			
1. Perform Procedure 7–1: Pre-Service—Preparing the Treatment Room.			
2. Place distilled water into the designated container through the fill opening in the top. Check that it is not too full and is level with the maximum fill line.			
3. Perform an equipment precheck and adjust the position of your equipment to ensure client safety and ease of use. Before beginning the facial, position the steamer where you want it. Adjust the height. Do not position the steamer arm/nozzle in the direction of the client. The steamer could sputter hot water onto the client. Wait until the steamer has demonstrated safe and effective steaming prior to directing on the client.			
4. Perform Procedure 8–1: Pre-Service—Prepare the Client for Treatment.			
5. Apply a makeup-remover to an esthetics wipe or cotton round and remove makeup.			
6. Apply facial cleaner and massage into the skin.			
7. Remove the cleanser from the skin.			
8. Using 2" × 2" esthetics wipes or cotton rounds moistened with toner, remove any residue.			
9. Apply eye pads or goggles.			
10. Turn on the steamer. If the steamer has a secondary option of ozone or vapor, do not turn on the second switch until steam is visible.			
11. When the water is boiling and steam is visible slowly adjust the steamer arm close to the client.			
12. Keep the steam approximately 15 to 18 inches (37.5 to 45 centimeters) from the face. Place the steamer farther away, if necessary, so that it is warm but not too hot on the face. If placed too close, steam can cause overheating of the skin, possible irritation, or burning.			
13. Always check the client's comfort level and ensure even distribution of the steam on the face. If the steamer is positioned with the steam directed from below the nose and is too close for the client, try steaming from above the head. Reposition it as needed to get an even placement of steam across the face.			

14. Never leave the client unattended while steaming as the water can spray out and burn the client. Do not oversteam the skin. Steaming should last 5 to 10 minutes but should be adjusted for less time if needed.			
15. When you are ready to discontinue the steam, move the steamer away from the client then turn off the steamer.			
16. Continue with the next step in the facial or close out this procedure.			
17. Remove eye pads or goggles, apply moisturizer and sun protection.			
18. Perform Procedure 8–9: Post-Service Procedure.			
19. Perform Procedure 7–2: Post-Service Clean-Up and Preparation for the Next Client.			
B. Cleaning and Disinfecting the Steamer			
20. Add 2 tablespoons (10 milliliters) of white vinegar and fill jar to the top fill line with water.			
21. Turn on the steamer and let it heat to steaming. Do not turn on the ozone.			
22. Let the machine steam for 20 minutes or until the water level is low, but make sure it stays above the bottom low-level line to avoid jar breakage.			
23. Turn off the steamer and let the vinegar solution rest in the unit for 15 minutes. Because vinegar has a pungent smell, clean the steamer in your utility room or in an area away from the treatment rooms. Open a window, if possible, when performing maintenance to keep fumes from traveling to other areas of the salon.			
24. After it cools, drain the steamer jar completely and then refill with water. Let the steamer heat to steaming again and operate for approximately 10 minutes. If there is still an odor, drain the unit and repeat the process.			

PROCEDURE 10–2: PERFORM DESINCRUSTATION AND IONTOPHORESIS USING THE GALVANIC MACHINE

Evaluate your practical skills.

CRITERIA	COMPETENT	NEEDS WORK	IMPROVEMENT PLAN
Procedure			
1. Perform Procedure 7-1: Pre-Service—Preparing the Treatment Room.			
2. Perform Procedure 8-1: Pre-Service—Prepare the Client for Treatment.			

3. Apply a makeup-remover to an esthetics wipe or cotton round and remove makeup.			
4. Apply a cleanser to the skin.			
5. Massage the cleanser into the skin to loosen makeup.			
6. Remove the cleanser from the skin.			
7. Using 2" × 2" esthetics wipes or cotton rounds moistened with toner, remove any residue.			
8. Cover the entire positive electrode that makes contact with the client with a piece of dampened cotton around the electrode. Give this to the client to hold or place behind the client's shoulder. This electrode is connected to the positive wire.			
9. Apply desincrustation fluid to the entire face and then apply the precut gauze face mask over the face.			
10. Apply the electrode to the client's forehead. Make sure the electrode is directly on the skin before turning on the galvanic current.			
11. Turn the switch to negative and set at the appropriate level for the client.			
12. Gently rotate the electrode while gliding it over the client's face. Do not lift the electrode or break contact once the machine is on the skin, or it will be uncomfortable for the client. Keep the electrode as flat as possible and parallel to the skin's surface at all times.			
13. Continue in the T-zone area down the nose and into the chin area (or into any area that is oily or needs desincrustation). Best practice is to use desincrustation only in congested areas that need it and avoid areas with dry skin conditions.			
14. Keep the electrode constantly moving to avoid overstimulating an area. Keep the skin moist. Add water to face if it gets too dry to glide over the skin.			
15. When you are finished, turn off the machine first and then remove the electrode. Rinse the skin thoroughly with moistened esthetics wipes.			
16. Continue with the next step; iontophoresis.			
17. Cover the entire positive electrode that makes contact with the client with a piece of dampened cotton around the electrode. Give this to the client to hold or place behind the client's shoulder. This electrode is connected to the positive wire.			
18. Apply ampoule or serum to the entire face and then apply the precut gauze face mask over the face.			
19. Dip the electrode into water or a conductive gel solution. Apply the electrode to the client's forehead. Make sure the electrode is directly on the skin before turning on the galvanic current.			
20. You have the option of switching positive and negative poles when infusing solutions. Consult the product manufacturer's instructions when doing so.			

	COMPETENT	NEEDS WORK	IMPROVEMENT PLAN
21. Beginning on the forehead, gently rotate the electrode while gliding it over the client's forehead. Do not lift the electrode or break contact once the machine is on the skin, or it will be uncomfortable to the client. Keep the electrode as flat as possible and parallel to the skin's surface at all times.			
22. Continue to the cheeks and the rest of the face.			
23. Keep the electrode constantly moving to avoid overstimulating an area. Keep the skin moist and the pads wet. Add water to the pad or face if it gets too dry to glide over the skin.			
24. When you are finished, turn off the machine first and then remove the electrode. Remove the gauze and rinse the skin thoroughly.			
25. Perform Procedure 8–9: Post-Service Procedure.			
26. Perform Procedure 7–2: Post-Service—Clean-Up and Preparation for the Next Client.			

PROCEDURE 10–3: USE THE HIGH-FREQUENCY MACHINE

Evaluate your practical skills.

CRITERIA	COMPETENT	NEEDS WORK	IMPROVEMENT PLAN
Procedure			
1. Perform Procedure 7–1: Pre-Service—Preparing the Treatment Room.			
2. Perform Procedure 8–1: Pre-Service—Prepare the Client for Treatment.			
3. Apply and massage a cleanser suitable to remove makeup into the skin with your gloved hands.			
4. Remove the cleanser using 4" × 4" esthetic wipes or chosen material.			
5. Using 2" × 2" esthetic wipes or cotton rounds moistened with toner, remove any residue.			
6. Apply the precut gauze face mask over the face, unless the electrode application listed later in this procedure does not require the gauze.			
7. Continue as noted with the appropriate electrode selection as detailed in Table 10–3 and proceed with the indicated steps listed for the specific electrode.			
8. Continue with the next step in the facial or close out this procedure with steps 11 through 13.			
9. Apply moisturizer and sun protection.			
10. Perform Procedure 8–9: Post-Service Procedure.			
11. Perform Procedure 7–2: Post-Service—Clean-Up and Preparation for the Next Client.			

PROCEDURE 10–4: USE THE SPRAY MACHINE

Evaluate your practical skills.

CRITERIA	COMPETENT	NEEDS WORK	IMPROVEMENT PLAN
Procedure			
1. Perform Procedure 7–1: Pre-Service—Preparing the Treatment Room.			
2. Perform Procedure 8–1: Pre-Service—Prepare the Client for Treatment.			
3. Apply and massage a cleanser suitable to remove makeup into the skin with your gloved hands.			
4. Remove the cleanser from the skin using 4" × 4" esthetic wipes or chosen material.			
5. Using 2" × 2" esthetic wipes or cotton rounds moistened with toner, remove any residue.			
6. If using the spray machine on a high setting you can place a towel under the client's chin to stop the mist from dripping down the neck. Turn on the power and adjust the velocity of the spray. Remind the client to keep the eyes and mouth closed during the misting.			
7. Hold the spray approximately 12 to 15 inches (30 to 37.5 centimeters) away from the face and mist for approximately 5 to 20 seconds. If necessary, pause and make sure the client can take a breath between the misting.			
8. Turn off the power.			
9. Perform Procedure 8–9: Post-Service Procedure.			
10. Perform Procedure 7–2: Post-Service—Clean-Up and Preparation for the Next Client.			

CHAPTER 11
HAIR REMOVAL

EXPLAIN THE IMPORTANCE OF HAIR REMOVAL

SHORT ANSWER

1. a) Melissa is expanding her spa and plans to move to larger location in order to have more space available for hair removal treatments. Why is this a good business decision?

_____

_____

_____

_____

_____

b) What is the most common hair removal method that Melissa could offer?

_____

_____

_____

_____

_____

DESCRIBE THE STRUCTURE OF HAIR

SHORT ANSWER

2. What is the scientific study of hair and its diseases called and why should you be knowledgeable about it?

_____

_____

_____

_____

_____

The Hair Follicle and Its Appendages

MATCHING

3. Match the descriptions to the terms.

a. follicular canal	c. hair papilla	e. arrector pili muscle
b. hair bulb	d. sebaceous gland	f. hair shaft

____ contracts when affected by cold or other stimuli

____ lined with epidermal tissue

____ part of the hair located above the surface of the skin

____ helps keep skin supple and waterproof with its secretions

____ cone-shaped elevation of connective tissue that contains capillaries and nerves

____ thick, club-shaped structure that forms the lower part of the hair follicle

List the Types of Hair

SHORT ANSWER

4. List and describe the three types of human hair.

- _____
  _____
  _____
  _____
  _____

- _____
  _____
  _____
  _____
  _____

- _____
  _____
  _____
  _____

EXPLAIN THE HAIR GROWTH CYCLE

SHORT ANSWER

5. Monica uses the acronym ACT to remember the hair growth cycle. Name and describe what happens during the three phases, noting which one is most important for the esthetician in effective hair removal.

_____

_____

_____

_____

_____

_____

_____

_____

_____

_____

IDENTIFY THE CAUSES OF EXCESSIVE HAIR GROWTH

SHORT ANSWER

6. List four factors that can determine the density of a person's hair growth on the scalp, face, and body.

- _____

- _____

- _____

- _____

Hypertrichosis Versus Hirsutism

MATCHING

7. Match the statements to the type of excessive hair growth. Types will be used more than once.

a. hypertrichosis	b. hirsutism

_____ excessive hair growth on the face, chest, underarms, and groin

_____ can be treated esthetically, but there is no cure to address the cause

_____ may be caused by stimulation of male androgens at puberty, medications, illness, and stress

_____ genetically and ethnically inherited

_____ can be resolved by eliminating the causes of the condition

_____ excessive hair growth of terminal hair in the areas of the body that normally grow only vellus hair

_____ caused by excessive male androgens in the blood

Common Diseases, Disorders, and Syndromes Affecting Hair Growth

FILL IN THE BLANK

8. A _____ is a group of symptoms that, when combined, characterize a disease or disorder.

9. A _____ is pathological, like conditions caused by viruses and bacteria, with a series of signs and symptoms.

10. A _____ is an abnormality of function, like a birth defect or genetically inherited malfunction.

11. The most notable and prevalent syndrome relating to hair growth is _____, which presents with hirsutism, irregular menses, ovarian cysts, and obesity.

COMPARE TEMPORARY AND PERMANENT HAIR REMOVAL AND REDUCTION METHODS

SHORT ANSWER

12. What is the difference between temporary and permanent hair removal?

_____

_____

_____

_____

_____

Temporary Methods, Home and Professional

MULTIPLE CHOICE

13. Which of the following is a method of depilation?

    a. shaving

    b. sugaring

    c. waxing

    d. tweezing

14. Which of the following is NOT a method of epilation?

    a. threading

    b. tweezing

    c. sugaring

    d. all answers are methods of epilation

MATCHING

15. Match the descriptions to the methods. Methods will be used more than once.

a. tweezing	d. chemical depilatory	g. waxing
b. electronic tweezing	e. threading	
c. shaving	f. sugaring	

____ spread on the skin to dissolve the hair

____ pull hair out by the root one at a time

____ snags unwanted hairs in a twisted portion of thread and epilates them

____ the fine tip of the hair shaft is removed

____ active ingredients are alkaline

____ alternative for those with sensitive skin

____ alternative for removing dark, coarse hair on the face if client is sensitive to waxing

____ also known as banding

____ can be done with a two-handed method or a hand and mouth method

____ ancient method dating back to the Egyptians

____ radio frequency is transmitted down the hair shaft into the follicle area

____ molded into a ball and pressed onto the skin, then quickly stripped away

____ may cause folliculitis, pseudofolliculitis, and ingrown hairs

____ most common professionally offered hair removal method

____ hair can be wiped away

____ applied in soft or hard form

____ ancient method that began in the Middle East

____ used in both directions, with hair growth and against hair growth

Permanent Hair Removal and Reduction

FILL IN THE BLANK

16. _____ is the only proven method of hair removal recognized and given the designation permanent hair _____ by the U.S. Food and Drug Administration and the American Medical Association.

17. _____ and _____ have been given the designation of permanent hair _____ because the effectiveness is dependent on the levels of pigment in the hair and skin.

18. _____ utilizes direct current (DC) from the probe, which creates a chemical reaction of sodium hydroxide to cause decomposition of the follicle.

19. _____ uses alternating current (AC) that is applied and emitted from the probe, inserted into the follicle of the hair to be eliminated, to destroy the dermal papilla.

20. The third main modality of electrolysis, when a combination of the two other methods is applied alternately or simultaneously, is called the _____.

SHORT ANSWER

21. Cassie's client is considering a permanent hair reduction service. Her client, who has very light blonde hair, asks specifically about a laser treatment or an intense pulse light treatment. How should Cassie explain the differences between these treatments to her client? Should Cassie suggest electrolysis for this client instead? Why or why not?

_____

_____

_____

_____

_____

EXPLAIN WHEN TO USE HARD AND SOFT WAX METHODS OF HAIR REMOVAL

TRUE OR FALSE

22. Circle whether the following statements about waxing methods are true or false.

T F   Regrowth from waxing can feel stubbly.

T F   Estheticians use hard wax in larger areas, such as the back and legs.

T F   Estheticians use soft wax in smaller areas, such as the eyebrows, axillae, and bikini area.

T F   Wax formulas are made from rosins, beeswax, paraffin, honey, and other waxes and substances.

T F   Soft wax uses a strip for removal.

T F   Overheating the wax diminishes its effectiveness and may cause injury.

FILL IN THE BLANK

23. Beth's client wants her eyebrows waxed. Correctly number the 11 steps Beth will go through to administer a hard wax treatment.

_____ Dip the small applicator into the wax and scrape the underside, to avoid threads.

_____ Repeat on the other eyebrow.

_____ With protective paper on the head of the table, client should be in a semireclined position with hair and clothing protected. Wash and dry hands then put on gloves.

_____ Having agreed on the desired shape during the consultation, brush eyebrows and measure for start point, arch, and endpoint.

_____ Apply pretreatment in accordance with wax manufacturer's recommendations, which with hard wax may mean its complementary prewax oil.

_____ Immediately apply pressure to the area.

_____ Finish with aftercare by massaging eyebrows with a soothing lotion and brushing them.

_____ Cleanse area to be waxed should of makeup, facial oils, and pollutants.

_____ When wax looks opaque and maintains a fingerprint, flick up the grasping edge of the wax on the outer edge of the eyebrow. Holding the skin taut at the outer edge, pull quickly against the direction of growth as close to the skin as possible.

_____ Follow procedure for the glabella. Tweeze or trim any stray hairs.

_____ Stand behind client and apply wax with small spatula to entire area under the brow.

MATCHING

24. Match the descriptions to the correct waxing method. Methods will be used more than once.

a. hard wax	b. soft wax

_____ strong enough for use on hard-to-remove, coarse hair and where hair growth converges from multiple directions

_____ allows for *speed waxing*

_____ consistency of honey when melted and runs down and around every hair while adhering to the skin

_____ can be used with caution on individuals using glycolic or other AHA skin care

_____ most common method of hair removal

_____ available in blocks, discs, pellets, or beads

_____ area can be waxed a second time during the service, provided there is no irritation

_____ has a lower melting point

_____ can use blending technique

SHORT ANSWER

25. Tammy's client has come in for a facial and wants to have some hair above her lip waxed. At what point during the facial should Tammy wax her client?

_____

_____

_____

_____

_____

PROVIDE A THOROUGH CLIENT CONSULTATION FOR HAIR REMOVAL SERVICES

SHORT ANSWER

26. Tasha's spa has a very in-depth questionnaire for new clients. She would like to design a shorter intake form for her regular repeat clients. What should be included in this client assessment form?

- _____

  _____

- _____

  _____

- _____

  _____

FILL IN THE BLANK

27. Mark the following with an X if they are contraindications for waxing.

_____ Client has scheduled a tanning appointment for later in the day.

_____ Client has not shaven for about 12 days and hair is longer than ½ inch.

_____ Client used an exfoliating body scrub the night before the service.

_____ Client has several ingrown hairs in area to be depilated.

_____ Client has varicose veins.

LIST ITEMS NEEDED IN A WAX TREATMENT ROOM

COLLAGE

28. Create a collage that shows at least five different pieces of waxing equipment. Beneath the collage list if each piece of equipment is furniture, a multiuse essential, single-use, or consumable item.

MIND MAPPING

29. Using the central or key point of *hygiene and infection control*, map out how you can reduce the risk of cross-contamination.

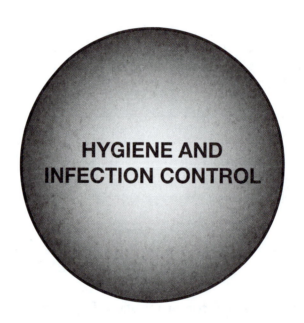

DEMONSTRATE WAXING HEAD TO TOE WITH SOFT AND HARD WAXES

MULTIPLE CHOICE

30. Hard or soft wax can be used on any part of the face or body except _____.

    a. chest   c. hands

    b. genitals   d. a man's beard

General Waxing Do's and Don'ts

SHORT ANSWER

31. List four general waxing do's and don'ts each.

    General Waxing Do's:

- _____

- _____

- _____

- _____

- _____

- _____

- _____

- _____

- _____

- _____

- _____
- _____
- _____

General Waxing Don'ts:

- _____
- _____
- _____
- _____
- _____
- _____
- _____

Face Waxing on Women and Men

LABELING

32. Max is about to wax a client's eyebrows. Mark the start, arch, and endpoint and how Max determined the placement using an applicator.

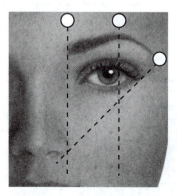

SHORT ANSWER

33. Max's next client is also getting an eyebrow wax. However, they have wider nostrils. How will Max adjust the applicator to get accurate start, arch, and endpoints?

_____

_____

Performing a Men's Eyebrow Wax with Soft Wax

SHORT ANSWER

34. Describe how a man's eyebrow waxing is different than a woman's eyebrow waxing.

_____

_____

_____

_____

_____

Waxing the Lip

LABELING/SHORT ANSWER

35. Draw the direction of hair growth on the upper lip. How are the hairs under the nose best removed?

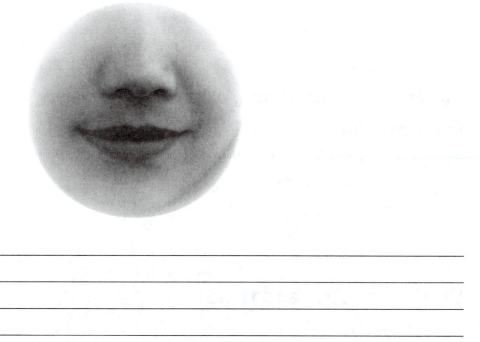

_____

_____

_____

_____

_____

Waxing the Chin

SHORT ANSWER

36. A new client has never had her chin waxed before and has only a few troublesome hairs. What should Ted tell the client when she requests to have her chin waxed?

_____

_____

_____

_____

_____

_____

_____

_____

_____

_____

Waxing the Sides of the Face

SHORT ANSWER

37. Your client Shannon is concerned about the hair on the sides of her face. You have explained the problems that waxing can create, but she is still determined. List two waxing methods you can offer to perform.

- _____
- _____

Waxing the Underarm (Axilla)

MULTIPLE CHOICE

38. When waxing the underarm, start _____.

   a. where there is the least amount of hair

   b. anywhere

   c. with the outside edge

   d. at the center

Waxing the Arm and Hand

FILL IN THE BLANK

39. _____ wax is the fastest, most effective way to remove hair on the arms.

40. If the hair is fine, it may be worth taking the time to remove the hair with _____ wax or _____, removing it with the growth and thus not distorting the hair follicles.

Waxing the Upper Body on Women and Men

MULTIPLE CHOICE

41. Before waxing upper body hair, trim it to _____.

    a. ¼ inch   c. ¾ inch

    b. ½ inch   d. 1 inch

Waxing the Chest

FILL IN THE BLANK

42. The female _____ should not be waxed.

43. Chest hair generally grows _____ in the décolleté, and across the chest and over the breast from the _____ toward the _____.

Waxing the Back

SHORT ANSWER

44. Ellen is about to begin waxing a client who wants his entire back waxed. Where should she stand while treating the client?

_____

_____

_____

_____

_____

Waxing the Lower Body on Women and Men

SHORT ANSWER

45. Describe the three types of bikini waxes.

    • Standard American bikini wax: _____

_____

_____

    • French bikini wax: _____

_____

_____

    • Brazilian wax: _____

_____

_____

WORD REVIEW

MATCHING

46. Match this chapter's vocabulary words with their definitions by filling in the correct letter.

_____ axilla	a. a modality of electrolysis combining alternating current (AC) and direct current (DC)
_____ blend	b. the hair on a fetus; soft and downy hair
_____ catagen	c. the border of the lip line
_____ depilation	d. the area between the eyebrows at the top of the nose
_____ epilation	e. second transition stage of hair growth where the hair shaft grows upward and detaches itself from the bulb
_____ glabella	f. scientific study of hair and its diseases and care
_____ hair papilla	g. cone-shaped elevations at the base of the follicle that fit into the hair bulb
_____ lanugo	h. longer coarse hair found on the head, face, and body
_____ syndrome	i. removes hairs from the follicles; waxing or tweezing
_____ terminal hair	j. professional and anatomical term for the underarm
_____ trichology	k. process of removing hair at the skin level
_____ vermillion border	l. a group of symptoms that, when combined, characterize a disease or disorder

DISCOVERIES AND ACCOMPLISHMENTS

In the space below, write notes about 10 key concepts discussed in this chapter. Share your discoveries with some of the other students in your class and ask them if your notes are helpful. Decide on the 5 most important concepts covered together. You may want to revise your discoveries based on good ideas shared by your peers.

Discoveries:

_____

_____

_____

_____

_____

_____

_____

_____

_____

_____

_____

_____

List at least three things you have accomplished since your last entry that relate to your career goals.

Accomplishments:

_____

_____

_____

_____

_____

_____

_____

_____

_____

_____

_____

EXAM REVIEW

MULTIPLE CHOICE

1. What is the final stage of hair growth?

    a. anagen

    b. catagen

    c. latent

    d. telogen

2. Jessica is opening a new salon and plans to dedicate much of the spa's square footage to hair removal services. Why is this a good idea?

    a. Current beauty trends favor hair removal.

    b. More estheticians are trained in hair removal treatments than in other treatments.

    c. Hair removal is a popular service that usually makes up a large part of a spa's business.

    d. Hirsutism is becoming increasingly common.

3. Which of the following is NOT an important part of hair removal procedures?

    a. room preparation

    b. safety

    c. infection control procedures

    d. timing the procedure

4. What is trichology?

    a. scientific study of hair-removal techniques

    b. scientific study of hair and its diseases

    c. technical term for mechanically removing hair

    d. technical term for artificially coloring hair

5. What is lanugo hair?

    a. fine, soft, downy hair

    b. short, coarse, shaved hair

    c. heavy, thick, strong hair

    d. hair found on the back and shoulders

6. Shelley's client has come in for facial waxing. The client prefers soft wax, but Shelley recommends using hard wax for which reason?

    a. The client has oily skin.

    b. The client has mature skin.

    c. The client uses skin care with glycolic acid.

    d. The client is also receiving a facial with extractions.

7. What is NOT a contraindication for facial waxing?

    a. recent cosmetic surgery

    b. recent reconstructive surgery

    c. recent laser treatments

    d. recent steam treatments

8. How long must virgin hair be in order to remove it with waxing?

    a. ¼ inch

    b. ½ inch

    c. ¾ inch

    d. ⅔ inch

9. What should clients avoid for at least 24 to 48 hours after waxing?

    a. moisture

    b. exercise

    c. salty foods

    d. excessive heat

10. When cleaning up the treatment room between clients, which step is not necessary?

    a. change table linens

    b. place tools in a disinfectant holding tray

    c. change wax heater collars if overly soiled with wax drips

    d. all steps are necessary

11. What happens to lanugo hair shortly after birth?

    a. replaced exclusively by vellus hairs

    b. replaced either by vellus hairs or by terminal hairs

    c. replaced exclusively by terminal hairs

    d. falls off, leaving those parts of the skin perfectly smooth

12. Tabitha's client asks for a bikini wax that leaves a small amount of hair on the front pubis area. What style of wax is the client requesting?

    a. American

    b. French

    c. Brazilian

    d. English

13. What is the acronym ACT used to help estheticians remember?

    a. procedural steps for a chin waxing

    b. safety steps for mechanical hair removal

    c. layers of the hair

    d. stages of hair growth

14. What is the anagen phase?

    a. the growth stage during which new hair is produced

    b. the transition stage of hair growth

    c. the final, or resting, stage of hair growth

    d. the dormant phase of hair growth

15. Pierre is about to perform a back wax on his client. The room is very small, and there is only room for Pierre to stand on one side of the table on which the client lies. How should Pierre approach the back wax?

    a. Pierre should complete the bottom of the back first for the client's comfort.

    b. Pierre should complete the top of the back first for the client's comfort.

    c. Pierre should complete the side of the back furthest from him first for his own comfort.

    d. Pierre should complete the side of the back closest to him first for his own comfort.

16. What is the second stage of hair growth?

    a. catagen phase

    b. anagen phase

    c. latent phase

    d. telogen phase

17. What is the function of a depilatory?

    a. permanently removing hair by extracting the root

    b. temporarily removing hair by extracting the root

    c. permanently removing hair by dissolving it at the skin's surface

    d. temporarily removing hair by dissolving it at the skin's surface

18. What is the removal of hair by means of an electric current that destroys the hair root?

    a. tweezing

    b. chemical depilation

    c. electrolysis

    d. epilation

19. Tim is setting up his wax treatment room. Which of the following disposable items will he stock?

    a. scissors

    b. bikini bottoms

    c. metal spatulas

    d. covered containers

20. Tim is also concerned about providing the proper aftercare for his clients. His wax treatment room should include which of the following for aftercare?

    a. witch hazel

    b. baby powder

    c. tea tree oil

    d. petroleum jelly

21. What shape is a hair follicle?

    a. club

    b. elongated triangle

    c. small sphere

    d. small tube

22. Estheticians should educate clients about the negative effects of waxing the _____.

    a. sides of the face

    b. upper arm

    c. underarm

    d. upper lip

23. What type of skin might benefit from sugaring as an alternative form of epilation?

    a. oily

    b. sensitive

    c. acne-prone

    d. Fitzpatrick IV–V

24. What direction is product applied during the hand method of sugaring?

    a. either with or against the direction of hair growth

    b. straight down on top of hair growth

    c. with the direction of hair growth

    d. against the hair growth

25. Cassie's female client has excessive hair growth on her face and chest. What might be causing this condition?

    a. genetics and ethnicity

    b. hyperthyroidism

    c. excessive male androgen production

    d. excessive estrogen production

26. What is NOT a form in which hard waxes are available?

    a. blocks

    b. pellets

    c. beads

    d. strips

27. What is true of soft wax?

    a. has a lower melting point than hard wax

    b. has a higher melting point than hard wax

    c. must be allowed to get tacky before removing

    d. must be applied thickly

28. When shaping an eyebrow for a client with a wide nose, where should the start point be for the placement of the applicator?

    a. alongside the nose, just above the nostril

    b. alongside the nose, just outside the outer nostril

    c. the tip of the nose

    d. the middle of the cupid's bow of the lip

29. For what purpose does an esthetician use pellon?

    a. wax formula ingredient

    b. threading

    c. chemical depilatory

    d. wax strips

30. What is the shape of the hair papilla?

    a. club

    b. tube

    c. cone

    d. round

31. What is the function of the hair root?

    a. infuses color into the hair

    b. lubricates the surrounding skin

    c. feeds nutrients to the hair

    d. anchors the hair to the skin cells

32. What is hirsutism?

    a. outgrowths of downy hair on body parts usually bearing terminal hair

    b. outgrowths of ingrown hairs causing skin irritation

    c. unusual hair loss on body parts

    d. excessive hair growth on body parts due to hormonal imbalance

33. What is the term for excessive hair growth in areas of the body that normally grow only vellus hair, and not necessarily in the adult male hair growth patterns?

    a. hypertrichosis

    b. carnauba

    c. hirsutism

    d. lanugo

34. Ken has a new client coming in for a hair removal treatment. Which of the following is an essential question that Ken should ask on the client's assessment form?

    a. How often do you shave?

    b. Do you ever tweeze unwanted hairs?

    c. Are you currently using any topical medications?

    d. Do you prefer soft or hard wax?

35. What is NOT true of laser hair removal and intense pulsed light (IPL)?

    a. effectiveness dependent on levels of pigment in hair and skin

    b. involves pulsing a laser on skin

    c. hair growth is impaired by this method

    d. several wavelengths used at one time

36. What is contained within the pilosebaceous unit?

    a. hair follicle

    b. arrector pili muscle

    c. sebaceous glands

    d. all of the above

37. What is an ancient method of hair removal?
    a. tweezing
    b. shaving
    c. chemical depilatory
    d. sugaring

38. Toni's client has requested a wax treatment on her upper arm, where there are only a few hairs just above the elbow. What technique should Toni use?
    a. electrolysis
    b. threading
    c. epilation
    d. blending

39. Carl's client, who has signs of hypertrichosis, asks if he can cure her condition. How might Carl respond?
    a. suggest that a doctor treat the client's excessive androgen production
    b. suggest depilation to permanently remove the hair growth
    c. recommend a hard wax treatment
    d. tell her that there may not be a cure for hypertrichosis, but it can be treated esthetically

40. When waxing the lip, where are there often nuisance hairs that bother the client?
    a. the vermillion border
    b. the glabella
    c. the axilla
    d. the areola

PROCEDURE 11–1: EYEBROW TWEEZING

Evaluate your practical skills.

CRITERIA	COMPETENT	NEEDS WORK	IMPROVEMENT PLAN
Procedure			
1. Discuss with the client the desired and appropriate shape.			
2. The head of the table should have protective paper for under the head, neck, and shoulders. The client should be in a semireclined position on the table, with the scalp hair protected and off the face. Wash and dry your hands then put on gloves.			
3. Cleanse and prepare the skin, using a makeup remover to remove makeup if present, otherwise using a mild antiseptic.			
4. With a disposable brush measure the start point, endpoint, and correct arch location.			
5. Brush the brows upward and isolate longer hairs that require trimming. Trim longer hairs with small round-tipped scissors to be uniform with the natural brow line. Brush along the top of the brow line and decide which hairs need to be removed.			
6. Standing or sitting behind the client and using the middle finger and forefinger, apply gentle friction to the brow area to warm the area, open the pores, and minimize discomfort during tweezing.			
7. Using the forefinger and middle finger of the hand not holding the tweezers, hold the skin of the brow taut. Remove unwanted hairs underneath the brow closer to the nose, working to the outer edge using a quick smooth motion, grasping the hair as close to the skin as possible without pinching it, and tweezing the hair in its direction of growth rather than pulling straight up.			
8. Brush the hair downward and remove hairs above the brow as necessary for the predetermined shape. After completing the brow, repeat the procedure on the second brow.			
9. Proceed to the glabella, the area between the brows, where some hairs grow upward and some downward.			
10. Wipe the treated area with a soothing, nonirritating antiseptic lotion to close the follicles and reduce the risk of infection.			
11. Finish by brushing the eyebrows in line.			

PROCEDURE 11–2: EYEBROW WAX WITH HARD WAX

Evaluate your practical skills.

CRITERIA	COMPETENT	NEEDS WORK	IMPROVEMENT PLAN
Procedure			
1. The head of the table should have protective paper for under the head, neck, and shoulders. The client should be in a semireclined position on the table, with hair and clothing protected. Wash and dry your hands then put on gloves.			
2. The area to be waxed should be cleansed of makeup, facial oils, and pollutants.			
3. Pretreatment should be in accordance with the wax manufacturer's recommendations, which may mean, with hard wax, its complementary prewax oil.			
4. Having agreed on the desired shape during the consultation, brush the eyebrows using a disposable brush. Measure the eyebrows for the start point, endpoint, and point of arch.			
5. Dip the small applicator into the wax and scrape the underside, to avoid threads.			
6. Standing behind the client, with a small spatula, apply the wax to the entire area under the brow, first against the direction of hair growth, and back over the same area in the direction of growth. Two or three applications may be necessary so that neither the hair nor the skin is visible through the wax. The strip of wax should have a clean, even edge all the way around for a clean removal, with a thicker tab at the outer edge where it will be lifted for the removal.			
7. Within 30 seconds, when the wax looks opaque and maintains a fingerprint it is ready to lift off. Flick up the grasping edge of the wax on the outer edge of the eyebrow and with a thumb, hold the skin taut at the outer edge. Grasp the wax and pull quickly against the direction of growth as close to the skin as possible.			
8. Immediately apply pressure to the area. Once you have become proficient in the use of hard wax, the wax can be applied to the second eyebrow while you are waiting for the wax on the first eyebrow to set.			
9. Repeat on the other eyebrow.			

10. When applying wax to the glabella, the area between the eyebrows, the procedure is the same—apply the wax first against the growth then back on top in the direction of growth and remove against the growth. Although there may be growth upward at the top of the glabella and downward at the top of the nose, hard wax can remove both directions in a single application and removal. Note: If needed, tweeze above each brow to remove any stray hairs. If needed, trim any extra-long stray hairs using rounded brow scissors.			
11. Finish with aftercare by massaging both eyebrows simultaneously with a soothing lotion and brushing the eyebrows.			

PROCEDURE 11–3: EYEBROW WAX WITH SOFT WAX

Evaluate your practical skills.

CRITERIA	COMPETENT	NEEDS WORK	IMPROVEMENT PLAN
Procedure			
1. The head of the table should have protective paper for under the head, neck, and shoulders. The client should be in a semireclined position on the table, with hair and clothing protected. Wash and dry your hands then put on gloves.			
2. The area to be waxed should be cleansed of makeup, facial oils, and pollutants.			
3. Pretreat the area to be waxed with the wax manufacturer's recommended products for soft wax or a thin film of tea tree oil followed by an application of baby powder.			
4. Having agreed on the desired shape during the consultation, brush the eyebrows using a disposable brush. Measure the eyebrows for the start point, endpoint, and point of arch.			
5. Dip the small applicator into the wax and scrape the underside, to avoid threads.			
6. Standing behind the client, glide the applicator at a 45-degree angle along the underside from the nose point to the outer edge, following the desired line for hair to be removed. For extensive reshaping of considerable hair, a tiny amount of wax on the applicator can be used to separate and pull hairs down and away from the brow line. This can be done facing the client, although the actual waxing is better achieved by standing behind the client.			
7. Then place the 1" × 3" strip over the wax, leaving a free edge at the endpoint to grasp. Give two or three quick strokes over the strip, also in the direction of hair growth.			

	COMPETENT	NEEDS WORK	IMPROVEMENT PLAN
8. Place the forefinger and middle finger at the endpoint, holding the skin taut, and pull the strip quickly back against the hair growth, as close to the skin as possible.			
9. Quickly apply gentle pressure with the fingers that held the skin taut.			
10. Repeat on the other eyebrow, and then the glabella. Following the rules for soft wax application and removal, the hairs higher up, growing upward, need to be treated separately from those at the top of the nose that grow downward. Note: If needed, tweeze above each brow to remove any stray hairs and trim any extra-long stray hairs using rounded brow scissors.			
11. Finish with aftercare by massaging both eyebrows simultaneously with a soothing lotion and brushing the eyebrows.			

PROCEDURE 11–4: PREFORM A LIP WAX WITH HARD WAX

Evaluate your practical skills.

CRITERIA	COMPETENT	NEEDS WORK	IMPROVEMENT PLAN
Procedure			
1. Complete draping and pretreatment preparations as outlined in Procedure 11–2.			
2. The area to be waxed should be cleansed of makeup, facial oils, and pollutants.			
3. Pretreatment should be in accordance with the wax manufacturer's recommendations, which may mean, with hard wax, its complementary prewax oil.			
4. Standing behind the client and using a medium-sized applicator, apply the wax to half of the upper lip, gliding up under the hair, against the growth, from the outer edge to the halfway point, under the septum of the nose, then back down in a figure eight motion. The hair may be removed either with the hair growth (if you don't want to distort the hair follicles) or against the hair growth. A thicker tab of wax should be formed at the end where the pull will originate.			
5. If also waxing the lower lip, for expediency, wax can be applied to half of the lower lip while the first application is setting.			
6. When the wax has lost its stickiness and wet shine, grasp the tab and remove the wax close and parallel to the skin. Then apply immediate pressure.			
7. Repeat on the opposite side of the upper lip (and lower if called for).			
8. Finish by using both hands to massage with a soothing aftercare lotion.			

PROCEDURE 11–5: PERFORM A LIP WAX WITH SOFT WAX

Evaluate your practical skills.

CRITERIA	COMPETENT	NEEDS WORK	IMPROVEMENT PLAN
Procedure			
1. Complete draping and pretreatment preparations as outlined in Procedure 11–3. The area to be waxed should be cleansed of makeup, facial oils, and pollutants.			
2. Pretreatment should be in accordance with the wax manufacturer's recommendations.			
3. Standing behind the client and using a medium-sized applicator, start under the septum of the nose and apply a thin layer of wax in a downward, outward direction. It is important to make sure that the area under the nostril is covered and that no hairs are missed on the edge of the nostril as well as the hair along the edge of the vermillion border, all while avoiding the lip.			
4. Immediately after the wax is applied, place the 1" × 3" strip over it, leaving enough of a free edge on the outside to grasp. Give the strip two firm rubs in the direction of growth.			
5. With your fingers holding the same outer edge of the lip taut and stable, grasp the strip and pull it quickly across the lip area in the direction opposite of growth, as close to the skin as possible, following through with a quick sweeping movement.			
6. Quickly apply pressure to the area with the hand that held the skin taut, to ease the smarting sensation common with this type of waxing in this area.			
7. Proceed to the other side of the lip.			
8. Finish with an application of soothing lotion.			

PROCEDURE 11–6: PERFORM A CHIN WAX WITH HARD WAX

Evaluate your practical skills.

CRITERIA	COMPETENT	NEEDS WORK	IMPROVEMENT PLAN
Procedure			
1. Complete draping and pretreatment preparations as outlined in Procedure 11–2.			
2. Decide how many sections of wax have to be applied to remove the hair under the jaw and down the throat based on sections of approximately no more than 2" × 3" and divide the area accordingly. Hair on the throat grows up toward the chin and from the center outward along the jawline. On the chin hair grows downward.			

3. Standing behind the client, by the top of their head, apply the wax with a medium spatula to the first section. For expediency wax can then be applied to another section as long as it is not immediately adjacent to the first application.			
4. Holding the skin taut, remove one or more sections in the direction of the hair growth and apply pressure immediately after the pull.			
5. Apply the wax in small sections below the curve of the jawline.			
6. Remove the wax. Due to the contours of the chin, this area should be waxed in small sections.			
7. If there is hair along the jawbone, it can be removed in a sideways fashion, similar to a lip wax, preventing the chance of follicle distortion.			
8. Finish with aftercare as previously instructed.			

PROCEDURE 11–7: PERFORM WAXING OF THE AXILLA WITH HARD WAX

Evaluate your practical skills.

CRITERIA	COMPETENT	NEEDS WORK	IMPROVEMENT PLAN
Procedure			
1. Complete the draping and pretreatment preparations, having the client lie flat on the table. If the axilla is deep, place a rolled-up towel bolster under the back directly under the axilla to be waxed.			
2. If the hair is long so that it curls over, it should be buzzed or trimmed to ½ inch in length. This will make the service more comfortable and easier to evaluate the different directions of hair growth.			
3. Make sure both axilla are thoroughly cleansed of perspiration and deodorant and are dry.			
4. Have the client raise the arm above the shoulder, placing the hand behind the head. They should then reach across the body with the other hand and move the breast tissue down and away.			
5. Apply the wax against the growth, getting underneath all the hairs growing in different directions first before going back over the top, forming a thicker tab at the end where the pull will originate.			
6. If three different applications are necessary, a second application can be done while the first is hardening, as long as it is not directly adjacent to the previous wax application and enough space is left in between for the third application.			
7. Have the client turn their face away from the axilla to avoid any chance of being hit during the swift removal of the wax.			
8. Apply immediate pressure to the area after each removal pull, to ease any discomfort.			
9. Apply aftercare of soothing lotion to the completed side before moving to the next side.			

	COMPETENT	NEEDS WORK	IMPROVEMENT PLAN
10. Complete the opposite side and finish with aftercare. Reassure the client that any blood spots are due to the fact that the hair was removed at the papilla, this is a sign of a successful epilation, and they will soon reabsorb into the skin. Ask the client to refrain from using deodorant on the area for at least 24 to 48 hours and until all signs of redness and irritation pass.			

PROCEDURE 11–8: PERFORM AXILLA WAXING WITH SOFT WAX

Evaluate your practical skills.

CRITERIA	COMPETENT	NEEDS WORK	IMPROVEMENT PLAN
Procedure			
1. Complete preparation, draping and positioning of client, and bolstering. To do this, have the client lie flat on the table. If the axilla is deep, place a rolled-up towel bolster under the back directly under the axilla to be waxed. Have the client raise the arm above the shoulder, placing the hand behind the head.			
2. If the hair is long so that it curls over, it should be buzzed or trimmed to ½ inch in length. This will make it more comfortable and easier to evaluate the different directions of hair growth.			
3. Clean the axilla on both sides thoroughly, removing any trace of perspiration and deodorant and pat dry.			
4. Ask the client to reach across their body and move the breast tissue down and away.			
5. With the edge of a large applicator, apply wax at a 45-degree angle in the direction of hair growth, where possible. If there are different directions within the same cluster, there could be breakage and some hairs left behind. As the same patch cannot be waxed a second time during that service, the remaining hair needs to be tweezed.			
6. Using a 3" × 9" wax removal strip, place the strip of wax and rub two times in the direction of growth. Instruct the client to turn their head away to avoid being hit and pull against the hair growth and close to the skin.			
7. Each application should proceed by clearing the outer edges working toward the center until the hair has been removed.			
8. Apply aftercare of soothing lotion to the completed side before moving to the next side.			
9. Evaluate the directions of growth on the second axilla as they may well be different than the first, this is more pertinent to soft waxing than hard waxing.			
10. Complete the wax application and removal on the opposite side and finish with aftercare as instructed in Procedure 11–8, step 8. As the same patch cannot be waxed a second time during that service, the remaining hair needs to be tweezed.			

PROCEDURE 11–9: PERFORM ARM AND HAND WAXING WITH HARD WAX

Evaluate your practical skills.

CRITERIA	COMPETENT	NEEDS WORK	IMPROVEMENT PLAN
Procedure			
1. Have the client sit on the side of the table and remove clothing from arms, exposing the area to be waxed. Complete draping by offering a disposable plastic apron or placing a drape across the client's lap and apply the pretreatment for hard wax.			
2. The first arm to be waxed is outstretched with the palm facing up. Start by waxing the inside lower half of the arm where there is less hair downward toward the wrist following the application rules for hard wax.			
3. The removal pull can be in the direction of growth if the goal is to not distort the hair follicles.			
4. The next section to wax should be just above the previous section.			
5. After completing the inner arm have the client turn their still outstretched arm, so the palm faces down. Then hold the arm firmly in place and, starting at the wrist, apply the wax across the top of the arm from the inside (thumb side) to the outside (little finger side), leaving the width of a strip between each application all the way up the forearm to the elbow.			
6. After removing the wax go back and wax those in-between sections.			
7. Next have the client hold their arm straight up, bent at the elbow, to wax the side that follows down from the little finger. This can be done in two sections starting near the elbow, working up toward the wrist. The hair grows down toward the elbow. Remove the wax.			
8. For the upper arm, ask the client to relax the arm and allow the forearm to rest on the lap. Apply the wax in alternating sections, starting toward the elbow and working up toward the shoulder.			
9. After removing those sections of hard wax, apply the wax to the remaining in-between sections. Remove the wax. If waxing only the arm, apply aftercare.			
10. To continue to the hand wax, ask the client to form a fist by tucking the fingers under, as this tightens the skin.			
11. Apply the wax, down toward the fingers, angling out slightly toward the little finger. The entire top of the hand can be done at once.			
12. To remove the wax, since the client's hand is "floating" without solid support, it is important to have a good grip on the hand for the removal pull.			

13. If the fingers need waxing, as the hair grows in a horseshoe shape, the hard wax can be applied in circular patches on each finger starting with the thumb across to the little finger.			
14. Once each finger application is completed, you will be ready to remove the wax in the same order.			
15. Apply aftercare by grasping the hand and applying the soothing lotion in long strokes up to the elbow and back down to the hand followed by a hand and finger massage. Proceed to the second arm.			

PROCEDURE 11–10: PERFORM ARM AND HAND WAXING WITH SOFT WAX

Evaluate your practical skills.

CRITERIA	COMPETENT	NEEDS WORK	IMPROVEMENT PLAN
Procedure			
1. Have the client sit on the side of the table and remove clothing from arms, exposing the area to be waxed. Complete draping by offering a disposable plastic apron or placing a drape across the client's lap.			
2. Apply the pretreatment for soft wax.			
3. With the client holding the arm outstretched with the palm facing up, start by waxing hair on the inside of the lower half of the arm, toward the wrist, where there is less hair. The hair grows downward toward the wrist, so the wax is applied following the growth and is removed against the growth.			
4. Apply the wax strip and rub firmly two times in the direction of hair growth. Hold the skin taut and remove the wax strip in one quick pull. The next section to wax should be just above the previous section.			
5. Next the client should turn their still outstretched arm so the palm faces down. Then hold the arm firmly in place and start at the wrist, applying the wax the width of the strip across the top of the arm from the inside (thumb side) to the outside (little finger side). Follow the rules of application and removal.			
6. Continue in strip-size sections all the way up the forearm to the elbow.			
7. Next have the client hold the arm straight up, bent at the elbow, and apply the wax to the side that follows down from the little finger. This can be done in two sections. The hair grows down toward the elbow.			
8. For the upper arm, ask the client to relax the arm and allow the forearm to rest on the lap. Apply wax in the direction of growth, which is downward, toward the elbow. Remove the hair in sections starting toward the elbow and working up toward the shoulder, blending if necessary at the top. If waxing only the arm, apply aftercare.			

9. To continue to the hand wax, ask the client to form a fist by tucking the fingers under, as this tightens the skin. Apply the wax with the growth, down toward the fingers, angling out slightly toward the little finger. The entire top of the hand can be done at once, not including the fingers.			
10. Apply the strip over the entire area and rub firmly in the direction of growth. As the client's hand is "floating" without solid support, it is important to have a good grip on the hand when you pull quickly back against the growth. Apply pressure after pulling off the wax strip.			
11. If the fingers have hair that needs to be removed and it is minimal and soft, it can often be removed with the wax that is already on the strip. The hair grows toward the middle knuckle, so take one finger at a time, press the wax onto the hair, rub in the direction of growth, and quickly pull off against the growth.			
12. If the finger hair cannot be removed by pressing the wax-saturated strip, complete the process by starting at the thumb and applying wax to each finger, then quickly going back and removing it.			
13. Apply aftercare by grasping the hand and applying the soothing lotion in long strokes up to the elbow and back down to the hand followed by a hand and finger massage. Proceed to the second arm.			

PROCEDURE 11–11: PERFORM A MEN'S CHEST WAXING WITH HARD WAX

Evaluate your practical skills.

CRITERIA	COMPETENT	NEEDS WORK	IMPROVEMENT PLAN
Procedure			
1. Complete draping with the client undressed from the waist up and fully reclined. Trim hair that is longer than ½ inch.			
2. Brush away the trimmed hair clippings, cleanse the skin and apply the pretreatment for hard wax.			
3. Using a large applicator, apply the wax on the furthest lower outer edge of the area of the chest where there is minimal hair.			
4. For expediency, a second wax application can be done while waiting for the previous one to set, as long as it is not immediately adjacent.			
5. Remove the wax. Apply gentle pressure immediately after each pull in this sensitive area.			
6. Move in sections upward and inward. As you get to the denser areas be mindful of changes in the direction of hair growth and make sure that the hair is well coated in wax.			
7. After completing the furthest side, continue in the same manner on the nearest side, beginning at the lower outer edge with less hair.			

	COMPETENT	NEEDS WORK	IMPROVEMENT PLAN
8. Next turn your attention to the hair growing in a different direction in the center, again starting where there is less hair, usually lower on the chest, and moving toward more dense hair, usually in the center and higher up on the chest.			
9. After hair removal is complete, finish by applying and massaging a soothing wax removal lotion to the area and checking for blood spots before the client dresses. Remind the client that blood spots are normal where hair is coarse and grows deep and that they are a sign of a successful epilation, not a cause for concern.			

PROCEDURE 11–12: PERFORM A MEN'S CHEST WAXING WITH SOFT WAX

Evaluate your practical skills.

CRITERIA	COMPETENT	NEEDS WORK	IMPROVEMENT PLAN
Procedure			
1. Complete draping with the client undressed from the waist up and fully reclined. Trim hair that is longer than ½ inch.			
2. Brush away the trimmed hair clippings, cleanse the skin, and apply the pretreatment for soft wax.			
3. Using a large applicator, apply the wax on the furthest lower outer edge of the area of the chest where there is minimal hair. The application should be no larger than the 3" × 9" removal strip.			
4. Rub the strip in the direction of the hair growth and remove the strip against the growth and parallel to the skin. Apply gentle pressure immediately after each pull in this sensitive area.			
5. Move in sections upward and inward. As you get to the denser areas be mindful of changes in the direction of growth.			
6. After completing the furthest side, continue in the same manner on the nearest side, beginning at the lower outer edge with less hair.			
7. Next remove the hair growing in a different direction in the center, starting where there is less hair, usually lower on the chest, and moving toward more dense hair, usually in the center and higher up on the chest. Wax this area in smaller sections, paying attention to the most dominant direction of growth or switch to hard wax in those areas.			
8. After hair removal is complete, finish by applying and massaging a soothing wax removal lotion to the area and checking for blood spots before the client dresses. Remind the client that blood spots are normal where hair is coarse and grows deep and that they are a sign of a successful epilation, not a cause for concern.			

PROCEDURE 11–13: PERFORM A MEN'S BACK WAXING WITH HARD WAX

Evaluate your practical skills.

CRITERIA	COMPETENT	NEEDS WORK	IMPROVEMENT PLAN
Procedure			
1. Complete draping with the client undressed from the waist up and fully reclined face down. The face should be in a face cradle with a disposable cover or with the forehead resting on the hands with the elbows sticking out. For comfort, you could place a bolster or rolled towel under their feet.			
2. Cleanse and complete the pretreatment preparations for hard wax. While cleansing, familiarize yourself with the directions of hair growth on the client's back, the length of hair, and inspect the back for skin tags, moles, and lesions.			
3. If the hair is longer than ½ inch, it should be trimmed. Afterward, wipe away the trimmed hair with an esthetics wipe, and then apply a dusting of powder, or pretreatment recommended by the hard wax manufacturer.			
4. Using a large applicator, first apply the wax on the outer edge of the torso, just above the waistline where there is minimal hair. Apply the wax in a manageable strip of approximately 2" × 5", using the application rules for hard wax.			
5. For expediency, while the wax is setting another application can be made, not immediately adjacent to the first application but one section over.			
6. Remove the sections following the rules for hard wax removal. Immediately apply gentle pressure to the area.			
7. Go back to the in-between section for the third application. Then while it sets, apply the fourth application to the area immediately adjacent to the second application, and so on.			
8. Continue in this manner until the side is cleared, following the waxing rules and directional changes. Include the back of the shoulder, if requested.			
9. Repeat on the opposite side.			
10. Next wax the hairs growing down the center of the back, over the spine.			
11. Apply aftercare of antiseptic lotion to the area that was waxed to remove wax residue, using effleurage massage strokes and being careful not to extend beyond the treated areas, as there may be a few more hairs to remove at the top with the client sitting up.			
12. The client should sit up, facing you with their arms at their side and a drape on their lap so the rest of the shoulder area can be waxed. These sections are smaller, so wax one surface at a time to avoid waxing over a curve.			

	COMPETENT	NEEDS WORK	IMPROVEMENT PLAN
13. Make sure both sides are balanced and even. Waxing the front is considered a separate service (part of the chest wax). Apply aftercare to the remaining areas.			
14. After wax residue is removed, apply a cool compress soaked in a baking soda solution for a few minutes. Remind the client that it is not unusual for hives to develop in the waxed area and they will settle down within an hour or so. Applying a salicylic acid product to the area can help reduce redness and bumps. As the client cannot see the back, let the client know when the blood spots have diminished before getting dressed.			

PROCEDURE 11–14: PERFORM A MEN'S BACK WAXING WITH SOFT WAX

Evaluate your practical skills.

CRITERIA	COMPETENT	NEEDS WORK	IMPROVEMENT PLAN
Procedure			
1. Complete draping with the client undressed from the waist up and fully reclined face down. The face should be in a face cradle with a disposable cover or with the forehead resting on the hands with the elbows sticking out. Waistband and undergarments should be protected with disposable towels.			
2. Cleanse and complete the pretreatment preparations for soft wax. While cleansing, familiarize yourself with the directions of hair growth on the client's back, the length of hair, and inspect the back for skin tags, moles, and lesions.			
3. If the hair is longer than ½ inch, it should be trimmed. Afterward, wipe away the trimmed hair with an esthetics wipe, and then apply a dusting of powder.			
4. Begin the hair removal at the area just above the waistline of the pants using a large spatula. The first application of wax should begin from the outside edge of the torso where hair growth is minimal.			
5. Follow the standard rules for soft wax application and removal. Grasp the strip, hold skin taut, and quickly pull parallel against the hair growth. Apply gentle pressure immediately after wax removal to ease any discomfort.			
6. The next application should be immediately above the previous one. If the length of the strip will be too long to do all at once, then apply a second strip next to the first. Remove the outside strip first, then the center.			
7. Repeat this process until you reach the top (toward the shoulders) as this is where you'll notice a change in hair direction. It begins to turn downward in the center along the spine.			

	COMPETENT	NEEDS WORK	IMPROVEMENT PLAN
8. Complete the removal on that side by following the waxing rules and directional changes. Include the back of the shoulder, if requested.			
9. Repeat on opposite side followed by the hairs growing down the center, over the spine.			
10. Apply plenty of soothing antiseptic lotion to the area that was waxed to remove the wax residue, being careful not to extend beyond the treated areas, as there may be a few more strips to do with the client sitting up.			
11. The client should now sit up, facing you with his arms at his side and a drape on his lap so the rest of the shoulder area can be waxed.			
12. The shoulders are waxed one surface area at a time. Do not attempt to round a curve with the strip. The hair on the shoulder usually grows inward to the center of the shoulder from the back, and inward toward the center from the front.			
13. Finish by blending toward the front and top of the arms, using existing wax on the strip and making sure both sides are balanced and even. Waxing the front is considered a separate service (part of the chest wax) but blending a little with wax already on the strip is acceptable.			
14. After all wax residue is removed, you can apply a cool compress soaked in a baking soda solution for a few minutes. Applying a salicylic acid product to the area will help reduce redness and bumps. Inform the client when the blood spots have diminished before getting dressed.			

PROCEDURE 11–15: PERFORM AN AMERICAN BIKINI WAXING WITH HARD WAX

Evaluate your practical skills.

CRITERIA	COMPETENT	NEEDS WORK	IMPROVEMENT PLAN
Procedure			
1. Complete draping by providing the client with disposable bikini bottoms or protecting the client's own undergarments with paper drapes. The client should lay face up flat or semireclined. Cleanse the area to be waxed.			
2. With an applicator select the hair to be removed, forming clean, even margins on both sides and keeping hair not to be removed securely tucked away and protected from the wax.			
3. If the hair is longer than ½ inch, it should be trimmed.			
4. Apply the pretreatment for hard wax.			

5. Ask the client to place the sole of the other foot to the level of the knee on the straight leg. The client should place one hand firmly on the paper or disposable panties on the pubis, fingers straight down. The other hand is placed on the outer edge of the thigh of the bent leg to help pull the skin taut. The hands and bent leg are reversed for waxing the opposite side.			
6. With a large applicator, apply the wax following the panty line up to the femoral ridge in a wax strip 2 inches wide and 4 to 5 inches long. Follow the rules for hard wax application, leaving a thicker tab at the end nearest the femoral ridge to grasp for the removal pull. If this area of hair is wide, it may take two parallel applications, so begin on the outer edge and work inward.			
7. Remove the wax, following the rules for hard wax removal and immediately applying pressure to the area after the removal pull.			
8. The next application is downward from the ridge toward the table, leaving enough space for hand placement to hold the skin taut. To facilitate this procedure, have the client bring the sole of their foot a little higher to just above the knee.			
9. Next have the client lift their leg to their chest, grasping it behind the knee or drawing it across the abdomen holding it by the ankle. This should expose the last remaining third of hair that was too near the table to apply the wax. This position also ensures that the skin is nice and taut.			
10. Apply the wax initially upward coating the underside of the hair then back downward over the top of the hair.			
11. The removal pull for this application is upward. When the first side is completed, continue on the other side.			
12. Apply soothing aftercare and remind the client that blood spots are normal and acceptable in this area, and a visible sign of a successful epilation.			

PROCEDURE 11–16: PERFORM AN AMERICAN BIKINI WAXING WITH SOFT WAX

Evaluate your practical skills.

CRITERIA	COMPETENT	NEEDS WORK	IMPROVEMENT PLAN
Procedure			
1. Complete draping by providing the client with disposable bikini bottoms or protecting the client's own undergarments with paper drapes. The client should lay face up flat or semi-reclined.			
2. With an applicator select the hair to be removed, forming clean even margins on both sides and keeping hair not to be removed securely tucked away and protected from the wax. If the hair is longer than ½ inch, it should be trimmed.			

3.	Cleanse and apply the pretreatment for soft wax.			
4.	Starting with the side furthest away have the client place the sole of the other foot to the level of the knee on the straight leg. The client should place one hand firmly on the paper or disposable panties on the pubis, fingers straight down. The other hand is placed on the outer edge of the thigh of the bent leg to help pull the skin taut. The hands and bent leg are reversed for waxing the opposite side.			
5.	With a large applicator, apply the wax following the panty line up to the femoral ridge in a wax strip 2 to 3 inches wide and 4 to 6 inches long following the rules for soft wax application. If this area of hair is wide, it may take two parallel applications, so begin on the outer edge and work inward.			
6.	Remove, following the rules for soft wax removal and immediately applying pressure to the area after the removal pull.			
7.	The next application is downward from the ridge toward the table, leaving enough space for hand placement to hold the skin taut. To facilitate the process, have the client bring the sole of their foot a little higher to just above the knee.			
8.	Next have the client lift their leg to their chest, grasping it at the ankle or behind the knee. This should expose the last remaining third of hair that was too near the table to apply the wax. This position also ensures that the skin is nice and taut. The soft wax is applied downward.			
9.	The removal pull for this application is upward.			
10.	When the first side is completed, continue on the other side.			
11.	Apply soothing aftercare and remind the client that blood spots are normal and acceptable in this area, and a visible sign of a successful epilation.			

PROCEDURE 11–17: PERFORM A LEG WAXING USING SOFT WAX

Evaluate your practical skills.

CRITERIA	COMPETENT	NEEDS WORK	IMPROVEMENT PLAN
Procedure			
1. Complete draping with client disrobed from the waist down and fully reclined on the table with legs stretched out and flat. If the feet and toes are to be waxed along with the legs, make sure they are kept warm with socks or a towel until ready to be waxed, or the wax will remain behind and not lift off with the strip.			
2. To pretreat the legs, mist the entire front area to be waxed with an antiseptic lotion then dust the entire area with baby powder.			

3. Have the client bend the knees and place the soles of the feet on the table. Then apply the mist and powder as far underneath as possible. For speed, prepare both legs simultaneously.			
4. Begin with the leg and foot furthest away if you have to lean rather than switch sides. Give the foot a good rub with both hands until it feels warm. Apply the wax to the top of the foot, applying it downward toward the toes.			
5. Apply the strip before the wax cools and pull off quickly as close to the skin as possible. Immediately apply pressure to the area.			
6. If there is very little hair on the toes, the wax on the strip may be sufficient to remove those hairs by pressing the wax onto the hair and quickly pulling away, making sure that the pressure is in the direction of growth, and the pull is in the opposite direction. If there is considerable hair growth, apply the wax to each toe.			
7. Rotate the foot outward. The next application is on the inside of the ankle. Apply the wax downward toward the ankle beginning from 7 to 8 inches up the leg. Continue with the next application directly above the previous one. Proceed in the same manner until the knee is reached.			
8. Rotate the foot back to the center and return. Then proceed again from the bottom, working in the same size strips, on the front of the leg up the shin bone to the knee.			
9. Rotate the foot inward. Starting again at the bottom, clear the hair in the same size strips to the outer edge of the lower leg, again working up to the knee.			
10. To wax the knees, have the client bend the leg and put the foot flat on the table. This area has coarse patches of dry, dead skin cells as well as folds of skin on some clients. This positioning ensures that the skin is tight. Apply the wax in downward, outward sections from the middle of the knee, covering the lower half.			
11. Apply the strip, rub firmly downward, and remove quickly upward, working your way around the knee.			
12. Next apply the wax to the top part of the knee in a downward direction over the top to the middle. Remove the wax strip.			
13. Next move to the upper leg. If the upper leg is not going to be waxed, you are ready to move to the other leg. The direction of hair growth on the upper leg is downward in the middle and outward on either side. Lay the leg back down and have the client rotate the foot inward for easy access. Apply the wax just above the knee to the center outward.			
14. Continue removing the hair by applying the wax from the center outward, moving up the thigh. It is especially important to hold the skin taut for the pull on the thigh, as the skin is often looser here than on the lower leg.			

15. Rotate the leg back to the middle and apply the wax in a downward direction from 8 inches above the knee downward toward the knee.			
16. After the middle is cleared, to wax the inner thigh, have the client bend the leg, bringing it to the same position it would be in if getting a bikini wax with the sole of the foot resting at the level of the knee on the other leg. Begin just above the knee, applying the wax from the inside down the inner thigh, leaving enough room near the table to hold the skin taut for the removal pull. Complete the inner thigh up to the bikini area, but not including the bikini unless that is part of this service.			
17. Next have the client grasp the ankle or under the knee, pulling the leg to the chest to expose the hairs at the back of the thigh while tightening that skin for comfort and effective removal. Be sure the skin is held as taut as possible to prevent bruising. An additional dusting of baby powder may be warranted.			
18. After completing the back of the thigh, move to the opposite leg, removing the hair in the same manner as on the first side.			
19. When the hair removal of the second leg is completed, lotion should be applied to the waxed areas to remove any residue so that the client does not stick to the paper when she turns over. This can be done with both hands simultaneously.			
20. The client now turns over for the remaining hair removal on the back of the legs. Have the client hang her feet off the end of the table and add an additional dusting of powder if necessary.			
21. Begin at the bottom of the lower leg and apply wax over the calf from the outside inward, continuing up in the same manner to the back of the knee.			
22. The hair growth pattern can vary at the back of the knee and should be determined at the time of waxing. Look for any patches of hair missed on the back of the thigh.			
23. When all the hair has been removed from both legs, pamper the client by applying plenty of lotion and using gentle effleurage movements, massage and sooth the legs with upward movements up the middle and a little lighter stroking down the outside.			

CHAPTER 12
MAKEUP ESSENTIALS

EXPLAIN MAKEUP ESSENTIALS AS IT RELATES TO AN ESTHETICIAN'S SKILLSET

SHORT ANSWER

1. Explain the importance of having a thorough understanding of makeup as an esthetician.

_____

_____

_____

_____

_____

_____

_____

_____

_____

_____

_____

DESCRIBE THE PRINCIPLES OF COSMETIC COLOR THEORY

SHORT ANSWER

2. Explain how understanding color theory can help you provide your client with an effective and pleasing makeup application.

_____

_____

_____

_____

_____

_____

_____

_____

_____

_____

The Color Wheel

DRAWING

3. Using markers, crayons, or colored pencils, create your own color wheels showing the primary colors, secondary colors, and tertiary colors. After completing your color wheels, label where the complementary colors and analogous colors appear.

FILL IN THE BLANK

4. Color _____ refers to the pureness of a color or the dominance of hue in a color.

5. Desaturated colors are colors mixed with white and located toward the _____ ring of the color wheel.

6. Desaturated colors are often considered _____.

7. The value, or _____, of a color is how light or dark it is.

8. The various degrees of _____ create tints, shades, and tones.

9. A tint occurs when _____ is added to a pure hue.

10. A shade occurs when _____ is added to a pure hue.

11. A tone occurs when _____ is added to a pure hue.

12. Colors with a yellow undertone and that range from yellow and gold through the oranges, red-oranges, most reds, and even some yellow-greens are known as _____ colors.

13. Colors that have a blue undertone, suggest coolness, and are dominated by blues, greens, violets, and blue-reds are known as _____ colors.

14. _____ colors do not complement or contrast any other color such as brown and gray, and earthy tones.

USE COLOR THEORY TO CHOOSE AND COORDINATE MAKEUP COLOR SELECTION

FILL IN THE BLANK

15. The three main factors to consider when choosing makeup colors for a client include

_____ , _____ , and _____ .

16. The tone of the skin is used to describe the warmth or coolness of a color and is generally classified

as _____ , _____ , or _____ .

17. For ruddy skin, apply a _____ - or _____ -tinted foundation to affected areas, blending carefully.

18. Use a _____ -based foundation to neutralize excess red in skin.

19. For sallow skin, apply a _____ -based foundation on the affected areas and avoid using _____ -based colors for eyes, cheeks, and lips.

Determine Eye Color

COLLAGE

20. Create a collage of different eye colors clipped from magazines. For those wearing eyeshadow, note which colors really make the eye colors pop. For those that do not have eyeshadow present, add complementary colors using crayons, colored pencils, or colored markers. Be sure to play with both light and dark shades as well as pure colors.

MIND MAPPING

21. Create a mindmap for determining all of the areas that you will need to evaluate before creating your client's color story. Begin with your client as the central circle then create branches such as your client's specific features and the types of products and colors that you will use.

Mature and Textured Skin

SHORT ANSWER

22. What are two tips that will help you select makeup for clients with textured and sun-damaged skin?

- _____
  _____

- _____
  _____

IDENTIFY FACE SHAPES AND PROPORTIONS FOR MAKEUP APPLICATIONS

SHORT ANSWER

23. Why is it important for a makeup artist to understand different face shapes?

_____

_____

_____

_____

_____

MATCHING

24. Match the face shape with its description.

a. oval	b. round	c. square	d. rectangle
e. triangle	f. heart	g. diamond	

The _____ face shape has well-proportioned features and is divided into three equal horizontal sections.

The _____ face shape is widest at the cheekbones. This face has a narrow chin and forehead.

This _____ face has a wide, angular jawline and forehead; the lines of this face are straight and angular.

Like a pyramid, the _____ face is widest at its base or jawline, tapering up to slightly narrower cheeks and reaching its apex at a narrow forehead.

The _____ face shape is long and narrow; the cheeks are often hollowed under prominent cheekbones.

The _____ facial shape is wide at the temple and forehead area and tapers down to a narrow chin, forming an inverted triangle.

The _____ face is widest at the cheekbone area and is usually not much longer than it is wide, having a softly rounded jawline, short chin, and rounded hairline over a rather full forehead.

DESCRIBE THE DIFFERENT TYPES OF COSMETICS AND THEIR USES

MATCHING

25. Match the product with its proper description.

a. foundation	b. primer	c. mineral makeup
d. concealer	e. face powder	f. blush
g. highlighter	h. eyeshadow	i. eyeliner
j. eyebrow color	k. mascara	l. makeup remover
m. lip color	n. lip liner	

_____ used to emphasize the eyes; pencil is the most commonly used form

_____ applied to the cheeks to give the face a natural-looking glow; helps create facial balance

_____ considered more noncomedogenic (less likely to clog pores) and natural than liquid foundations

_____ intended to fill uneven areas on the outer edges of the lips to define their shape

_____ darkens, defines, and thickens the eyelashes

_____ used to help frame the face; available in pencil, pomade, and gel formulations

_____ accentuates and brings out features such as the brow bone under the eyebrow, the temples, the chin, and the cheekbones

_____ adds a matte, or nonshiny, finish to the face while enhancing the skin's natural color and diminishing excessive color and shine

_____ may be oil based or water based and is good for removing mascara and other products

_____ covers blemishes and discolorations and may be applied before or after foundation

_____ designed to go underneath foundation and other products to prepare the skin for makeup and to help keep the product on the skin

_____ used to accentuate and contour the eyes; can be matte or shimmer

_____ also known as base makeup; a tinted cosmetic used to even out skin tone and color, and to conceal imperfections

_____ may contain moisturizers and sunscreen to protect the lips

PREPARE THE MAKEUP STATION AND SUPPLIES FOR CLIENTS

DRAWING

26. Using the space below or on a separate sheet of paper as your makeup table, draw or write all of the supplies you will need to provide your client with a successful makeup application. You can also clip images from magazines to represent each of your items. Be sure to include all of your makeup products, makeup brushes, and disposables needed for this service.

FILL IN THE BLANK

27. _____ bristle brushes and wooden handles are porous and cannot be disinfected.

28. _____ brushes are ideal as they don't require disinfection.

FOLLOW INFECTION CONTROL REQUIREMENTS FOR MAKEUP SERVICES

SHORT ANSWER

29. What measures should you take to prevent product contamination when applying makeup to your client?

_____

_____

_____

_____

_____

_____

_____

_____

_____

_____

_____

_____

_____

_____

_____

_____

_____

FILL IN THE BLANK

30. How do you properly clean the following multiuse items?

- **Applicators:** _____

   _____

- **Pencils:** _____

   _____

- **Testers:** _____

   _____

- **Palettes and supplies:** _____

   _____

CONDUCT A THOROUGH MAKEUP CONSULTATION WITH A CLIENT

SHORT ANSWER

31. What are seven helpful questions to ask your client during the makeup consultation?

_____

_____

_____

_____

_____

_____

_____

_____

_____

32. Describe the difference between a makeup lesson and a makeup application.

_____

_____

_____

_____

_____

_____

_____

_____

_____

PERFORM MAKEUP APPLICATION TECHNIQUES

FILL IN THE BLANK

33. When correctly applied, _____ creates an even canvas for the rest of the makeup application.

34. Makeup should blend smoothly with no _____.

35. _____ colors are darker shades used to define the cheekbones and make features appear smaller.

36. _____ powder blends with all foundations and will not change color when applied.

37. Apply blush just _____ the cheekbones, blending on top of the bones toward the top of the cheeks.

38. When applying eyeshadow, a _____ color can be make the brow bone appear larger, a _____ color will even out the skin tone and can be applied all over the lid to create a smooth surface for the blending of other color, and a _____ color is deeper and darker than the client's skin color and is applied to minimize a specific area or add depth to a crease.

39. _____ is a technique using one or both hands positioned to avoid client injury, keeping your hands steady and the client safe.

40. Apply foundation and powder _____ in the direction of the hairs on the face for better blending.

SHORT ANSWER

41. Explain the importance of bracing and how to incorporate it into your makeup application process.

_____

_____

_____

_____

_____

_____

_____

_____

USE HIGHLIGHTING AND CONTOURING TECHNIQUES FOR BALANCE AND PROPORTION

SHORT ANSWER

42. What is the rule to follow when highlighting and contouring?

_____

_____

_____

_____

_____

43. What techniques could you use to reshape your client's wide-set eyes?

_____

_____

_____

_____

_____

_____

Eyebrows

SHORT ANSWER

44. Your client would like to reshape her full brows and make her lips look fuller. You determine that she has a round face shape and both thin upper and lower lips. What steps will you take to address her brow and lip needs?

_____

_____

_____

_____

_____

_____

PERFORM A PROFESSIONAL MAKEUP APPLICATION

LABELING

45. Describe what is happening in each of the following pictures.

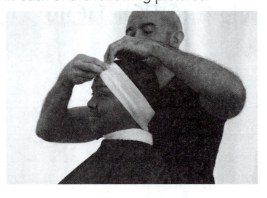

_____

_____

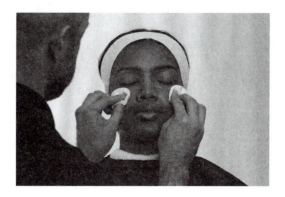

_____

_____

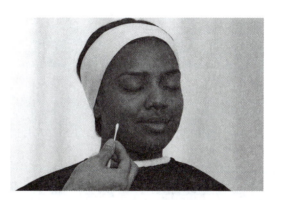

_____

_____

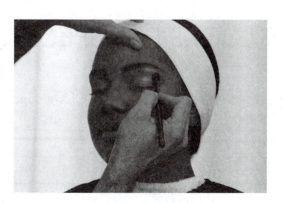

_____

_____

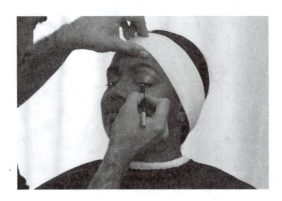

_____

_____

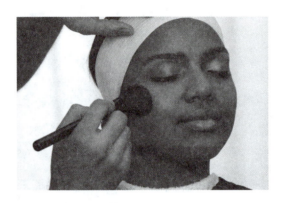

_____

_____

CREATE MAKEUP LOOKS FOR SPECIAL OCCASIONS

SHORT ANSWER

46. What are important considerations for makeup application for a special occasion?

_____

_____

_____

_____

_____

FILL IN THE BLANK

47. For the client looking for a specific bridal makeup, a _____ is recommended to help establish both the desired look, color preferences, and timelines for the day of the event.

APPLY MAKEUP FOR THE CAMERA AND SPECIAL EVENTS

FILL IN THE BLANK

48. Makeup formulated with photochromatic pigments that react with all types of lighting so the skin looks natural and flawless on camera is called _____.

SHORT ANSWER

49. How has HD changed makeup application?

_____

_____

_____

_____

_____

_____

_____

_____

_____

_____

RECOGNIZE THE BENEFITS OF CAMOUFLAGE MAKEUP

SHORT ANSWER

50. List some of the benefits of learning camouflage makeup as an advanced skill set.

_____

_____

_____

_____

_____

DEMONSTRATE THE APPLICATION OF ARTIFICIAL EYELASHES

FILL IN THE BLANK

51. The three types of artificial eyelashes are _____, _____, and _____.

52. List the contraindications that will prohibit you from providing your client with artificial lashes.

- _____
- _____
- _____
- _____
- _____
- _____
- _____
- _____
- _____
- _____

PERFORM THE APPLICATION OF ARTIFICIAL LASHES

FILL IN THE BLANK

53. Number the following steps in the preparation, procedure, and cleanup activities for applying artificial strip eyelashes in the order they should occur.

_____ Using a disposable brush, apply a thin strip of lash adhesive to the base of the lash and allow a few seconds for it to set.

_____ Prepare lashes. Brush the client's eyelashes to make sure they are clean and free of foreign matter, such as mascara particles. Curl the eyelashes with an eyelash curler before you apply the artificial lashes.

_____ Use tweezers to carefully remove the eyelash strip from the package.

_____ Lightly apply mascara to the tips to minimize separation between the false and natural lashes.

_____ Measure the strip lash by lightly placing them along the client's lash line. Shape eyelash. Adjust the length by trimming the outer edges of each strip.

_____ Apply the lash. Align the strip with the client's lash line, starting at the outer edge of the eye. Using an orange stick (wooden pusher) or the rounded edge of your tweezers to slide the strip right up to the base of the lashes.

DESCRIBE TINTING LASHES AND BROWS ON A MAKEUP CLIENT

SHORT ANSWER

54. What are some important tips to remember when tinting the lashes and/or brows?

- _____
  _____
- _____
  _____
- _____
  _____
- _____
  _____
- _____
  _____
- _____
  _____
- _____
  _____
- _____
  _____

FILL IN THE BLANK

55. _____ are single synthetic or natural hairs that are applied one-by-one to the client's natural lashes.

56. _____ is the process of chemically curling the lashes.

PERFORM THE TINTING OF LASHES AND BROWS

LABELING

57. Describe what is happening in each of the following pictures.

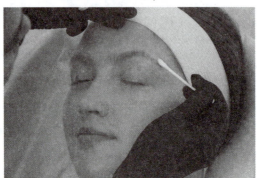

_____

_____

_____

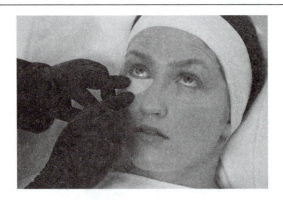

_____

_____

_____

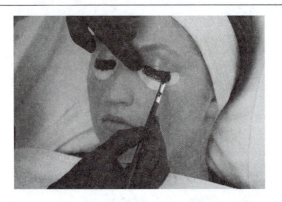

_____

_____

_____

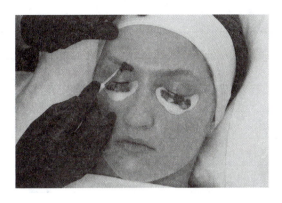

_____
_____
_____

DEFINE PERMANENT MAKEUP APPLICATION

FILL IN THE BLANK

58. _____ is a cosmetic implantation technique that deposits colored pigment into the upper reticular layer of the dermis; similar to tattooing.

59. The specialized techniques used for permanent cosmetics are often referred to as _____, _____, or _____.

60. _____ is defined as is a tattooing or semipermanent makeup technique where a small hand-held device, made up of tiny needles is used to add pigment to the skin.

DESCRIBE THE BENEFITS OF A CAREER IN MAKEUP

SHORT ANSWER

61. List some of the opportunities available to makeup artists and how you can promote yourself effectively.

- _____
_____
- _____
_____
- _____
_____
- _____
_____

- _____
  _____
- _____
  _____
- _____
  _____
- _____
  _____
- _____
  _____
- _____
  _____
- _____
  _____
- _____
  _____

PROMOTE RETAIL SERVICES AS A MAKEUP ARTIST

SHORT ANSWER

62. What should you consider when choosing a makeup line to retail?

_____
_____
_____
_____
_____

WORD REVIEW

FILL IN THE BLANK

63. _____ colors are located directly next to each other on the color wheel.

_____ is a technique using one or both hands positioned to avoid client injury, keeping your hands steady and the client safe.

_____ colors are primary and secondary colors opposite one another on the color wheel.

_____ colors have a blue undertone that suggest coolness and are dominated by blues, greens, violets, and blue-reds.

_____ refers to makeup colors that are darker shades used to define the cheekbones and make features appear smaller.

_____ is the metal part that holds makeup brushes intact.

_____ is a tinted cosmetic used to cover or even out skin tone and coloring of the skin.

_____ are lighter than the skin color; accentuate and bring out features such as the brow bone under the eyebrow, the temples, the chin, and the cheekbones.

_____ is any color in its purest form, lacking any black (shade) or white (tint).

_____ colors do not complement or contrast any other color; examples include brown and gray, along with multiple variations of each.

_____ colors include yellow, red, and blue.

_____ refers to skin that is red, wind burned, or affected by rosacea.

_____ refers to skin that has a yellowish hue.

_____ refers to the pureness of a color or the dominance of hue in a color.

_____ colors are obtained by mixing equal parts of two primary colors.

_____ refers to degree of saturation; occurs when black is added to a pure hue.

_____ colors are intermediate colors achieved by mixing a secondary color and its neighboring primary color on the color wheel in equal amounts.

_____ refers to degree of saturation; occurs when white is added to a pure hue.

_____ is used to describe the warmth or coolness of a color; generally classified as light, medium, or dark.

_____ is a color on which another color has been imposed and which can be seen through the other color.

_____ is also known as brightness of a color; how light or dark it is, which depends on the amount of light emanating from the color.

_____ colors include the range of colors with yellow undertones; from yellow and gold through oranges, red-oranges, most reds, and even some yellow-greens.

DISCOVERIES AND ACCOMPLISHMENTS

In the space below, write notes about key concepts discussed in this chapter. Share your discoveries with some of the other students in your class and ask them if your notes are helpful. You may want to revise your discoveries based on good ideas shared by your peers.

Discoveries:

_____

_____

_____

_____

_____

_____

_____

_____

_____

_____

_____

List at least three things you have accomplished since your last entry that relate to your career goals.

Accomplishments:

_____

_____

_____

_____

_____

_____

_____

_____

_____

_____

_____

EXAM REVIEW

MULTIPLE CHOICE

1. Sandra is setting up her makeup station. Where should the brightest light be coming from?

    a. directly overhead

    b. a window with natural light

    c. behind the client

    d. the light around the makeup mirror

2. What is one of the factors to consider when choosing colors for a client?

    a. skin type

    b. skin color

    c. natural lip color

    d. eyebrow color

3. How will you know if the foundation you've chosen for a client is the correct color?

    a. When applied, the color will blend in.

    b. When applied, the color will appear "sit" on top of the skin.

    c. When applied, the color will look artificial.

    d. When applied, the color will create a contrast between the face and the neck.

4. What is true of an eyeshadow base color?

    a. It is lighter than the client's skin tone.

    b. It is generally a medium tone close to the client's skin tone.

    c. It is deeper than the client's skin tone.

    d. It is only flattering to pale complexion tones.

5. What are colors with a blue undertone?

    a. cool colors

    b. primary colors

    c. secondary colors

    d. warm colors

6. You notice a client showing your colleague a picture of her wedding gown. How will this picture help determine the type of makeup to use?

    a. helps to determine timeline for the day

    b. helps to determine complementary colors

    c. helps to determine type of foundation to use

    d. helps to determine how formal the makeup should be

7. What coloration does sallow skin have?

    a. pinkish

    b. reddish

    c. greenish

    d. yellowish

8. How would you use highlighting and contouring to reshape a narrow face?

    a. apply a darker foundation over the chin and neck and a lighter foundation through the cheeks and under the eyes to the temples and forehead

    b. apply a darker foundation below the cheekbones and along the jawline; blend into the neck

    c. use two foundations, light and dark, with the darker shade blended on the outer edges of the temples, cheekbones, and jawline, and the light one from the center of the forehead down the center of the face to the tip of the chin

    d. blend a light shade of foundation over the outer edges of the cheekbones to bring out the sides of the face

9. One of your co-workers is on vacation and he has left you some notes on one of his clients. The notes tell you he creates width at the client's forehead and slenderizes her jawline. What is the likely face shape of the client?

    a. triangle (pear)

    b. rectangle

    c. round

    d. heart

10. You are a supervisor at a salon. As you are observing your staff, you see an employee opening a compact of pressed powder. What procedure should be used when removing the powder?

    a. use fingers to remove product

    b. have disposable gloves on

    c. use a new, disposable spatula to scrape the powder onto a clean palette

    d. use a tissue to wipe product from compact onto the client's skin

11. Clara has come in to get her eyebrows tinted; however, you determine that the treatment may not be effective. For what reason do you draw that conclusion?

    a. Clara has overplucked and the eyebrow hair is sparse.

    b. Clara's eyebrows are light blonde in color.

    c. Clara has oily skin.

    d. Clara also would also like to have a facial beforehand.

12. Michelle wants some suggestions on how to promote her services as a makeup artist. What should Michelle **NOT** do to promote her work?

    a. use social networking

    b. offer free makeup services to draw in customers

    c. create a professional portfolio to share with potential clients

    d. promote makeup services to facial clients

13. What is **NOT** one of the reasons estheticians should have a thorough understanding of makeup?

    a. Makeup knowledge can help to grow your clientele.

    b. Clients will rely on makeup artists for fresh and edgy looks.

    c. Color theory and facial analysis are part of being a successful makeup artist.

    d. Seasonal creation of new products is frustrating and confusing for clients.

14. What is **NOT** true of primers?

    a. They are liquid or silicone-based formulas.

    b. They are designed to go underneath foundations.

    c. They are designed to help foundation penetrate into the skin for blending.

    d. They prepare the skin for makeup and help keep product on the skin.

15. A client wants permanent eyebrow color. She's heard about microblading but doesn't know much about it. How would you explain microblading?

    a. It uses a small scalpel to insert pigment directly into the skin.

    b. It uses a series of needle injections which result in permanent color.

    c. It is semipermanent, requires touch-ups, and uses tiny needles.

    d. It cannot be done to the eyebrows.

16. Who often prefers liquid foundation over mineral makeup because mineral makeup can tend to be shiny and too dry?

    a. clients with dry skin

    b. male clients

    c. young clients

    d. mature clients

17. What is formed when white is added to a pure hue?

    a. tint

    b. shade

    c. tone

    d. saturation

18. Which of the following are benefits of airbrushing?

    a. It is water resistant.

    b. It is quicker to apply than traditional makeup.

    c. Neither a nor b is correct.

    d. Both a and b are correct.

19. Which face shape has long been considered the ideal?

    a. oval

    b. round

    c. diamond

    d. heart

20. Maria is attending a formal evening event. As her consultant, what makeup techniques will you suggest?

    a. eyeliner and eyeshadow in cool tones for both warm and cool skin tones

    b. darker eyeliner with a neutral lip color

    c. stronger look and false eyelashes

    d. palette of colors she normally uses and emphasize eyebrows

21. What are band lashes?

    a. small clusters of artificial lashes

    b. separate individual artificial eyelashes

    c. artificial lashes used in conjunction with heavy eyeliner

    d. artificial lashes on a strip

22. Which of the following are benefits of camouflage make-up?

    a. eliminates age spots and skin tags

    b. covers congenital issues and scarring

    c. restores overplucked eyebrows and enhances eyelashes

    d. gives an illusion of straight nose and symmetrical lips

23. Nancy wants a complementary color for her eyeshadow choice. Where on the color wheel is the complementary color located?

    a. directly next to each other

    b. one color removed from each other

    c. the same color, only different tints

    d. directly across from each other

24. A potential client wants to know if you have expertise with covering blemishes and discoloration. What would you use on this client?

    a. blush

    b. concealer

    c. highlighter

    d. contouring

25. What is **NOT** true of high-definition makeup?

    a. It blends into the skin to provide a flawless complexion.

    b. It contains photochromatic pigments to react with all types of lighting.

    c. It diffuses pores.

    d. It needs to be applied heavily.

26. What is attached to a client in the procedure called eye tabbing?

    a. band lashes

    b. mascara

    c. eyeshadow

    d. individual lashes

27. What kind of foundation diffuses imperfections?

    a. water-based

    b. alcohol-based

    c. silicone-based

    d. oil-based

28. What is greasepaint typically used for?

    a. glamorous evening look

    b. casual daytime look

    c. theatrical purposes

    d. pharmaceutical purposes

29. After determining skin tone, you are ready to apply foundation. How do you check for the correct shade and what in direction do you blend the foundation on the face?

   a. put small amount on forehead; blend downward

   b. put small amount on chin; blend outward and downward

   c. put small amount on highest part of cheekbone; blend outward

   d. put small amount on jaw; blend downward

30. Your classmate Rene is interested in pursuing theatre and film makeup artistry. She is aware that she _____.

   a. will have to operate her own makeup business for at least three years

   b. must take college credit courses to gain union membership.

   c. must be part of the stage crew or be cast in a play

   d. may need a lengthy apprenticeship and acceptance into a union

31. What is a short brush with dense bristles used for powder or blush?

   a. blush brush

   b. powder brush

   c. foundation brush

   d. kabuki brush

32. Tara is balancing the eye shape of her client who has round eyes. What technique will she use?

   a. blending dark shadow over the eyelid and carrying it toward the eyebrow

   b. using bright, light, reflective shadow colors

   c. applying concealer under the eyes and blending

   d. extending the shadow beyond the outer corner of the eyes

33. How are lash extensions applied?

   a. one-by-one to the client's natural lashes

   b. several at a time in clusters

   c. in groups of lashes using an adhesive

   d. over many appointments done in small sets as partials

34. After cleansing and rinsing brushes, how should you dry them?

   a. place upright, with bristles in the air, in a container

   b. lay flat in a closed, sealed container

   c. reshape the wet bristles and lay the brush flat to dry

   d. brush them briskly against a clean towel or new paper towel until dry

35. Which of the following would **NOT** be an appropriate infection control measure for applicators?

      a. disinfect applicators with sponge-tips for reuse

      b. use new spatulas to distribute products

      c. disinfect multi-use tools after each use

      d. do not double-dip applicators back into products

36. Permanent makeup is a cosmetic implantation technique that deposits colored pigment into what layer of the skin?

      a. reticular layer of the dermis

      b. stratum corneum of the epidermis

      c. stratum lucidum of the epidermis

      d. papillary layer of the dermis

37. You are an attentive esthetician who understands infection risk. What is an effective habit you can use to avoid spreading infection?

      a. washing your hands before you start a session

      b. using disinfectant wipes on your work table

      c. making sure your vaccinations are current

      d. using brushes with natural bristles

38. What is the term for colors that are formed by mixing equal amounts of a primary color and its neighboring secondary color on the color wheel?

      a. complementary colors

      b. secondary colors

      c. analogous colors

      d. tertiary colors

39. When applying mascara, what should you **NOT** do?

      a. use a side-to-side motion from the base to the tip of lashes for more coverage

      b. have the client look up at the ceiling when applying mascara to lower lashes

      c. dispose of each wand into a lined waste receptacle, being sure not to double-dip

      d. point the wand toward the eye when coating the tips of the lashes

40. What needs to be considered when choosing a makeup line to retail?

      a. the newest lines as their products have the latest research

      b. a line that is expensive as that means it is high quality

      c. a line that provides all the product displays to save you time

      d. a line you like working with and feel comfortable recommending

41. Your next client is self-conscious about her short, thick neck. Which makeup technique can give the illusion of elongating the neck?

   a. use a lighter color at the base of the neck

   b. use a lighter color down the center of the neck and a darker foundation on the sides of the neck

   c. use a lighter foundation along the jaw line

   d. use a darker foundation on the chin and base of the neck

42. Ruth would like to camouflage her double chin with makeup. Which technique should Dana use to reshape Ruth's face?

   a. highlight her cheekbones and feather upward

   b. shade under her jawline and chin

   c. use concealer along the length and center of her neck

   d. use a brighter lip color and a darker eyeliner

43. What is an example of a secondary color?

   a. blue

   b. white

   c. green

   d. blue-violet

44. During an initial consultation for makeup, your new client seems nervous about her answers and choices on the questionnaire. You assure her that besides the questionnaire, you can
   _____.

   a. keep trying different looks during the session

   b. use colors that are neutral so the questionnaire becomes unimportant

   c. show her various looks from magazines for inspiration

   d. go over the questionnaire again until she is confident

45. One of your clients is having professional photographs taken. Which of the following actions should you take to provide the best makeup possible for the photos?

   a. apply a translucent powder to keep makeup colors from running together under intense lighting conditions

   b. use darker colors for eyeliner and foundation and outline her lips in a darker lip color

   c. ask to see the makeup on a monitor to check color intensity

   d. ask to see the outfit she will wear for the session

PROCEDURE 12–1: PERFORMING A PROFESSIONAL MAKEUP APPLICATION

Evaluate your practical skills.

CRITERIA	COMPETENT	NEEDS WORK	IMPROVEMENT PLAN
Preparation			
Perform Procedure 7–1 and 8–1: Pre-Service Procedures.			
Start by setting out a few color selections: neutrals, cools, warms.			
The client's skin needs to be exfoliated and hydrated for the makeup to be applied successfully. This should happen before the procedure, but if there is extra time the client can wash and exfoliate their face at a sink. You might ask them to come in early for this.			
Procedure			
1. Determine the client's needs, choosing products and colors accordingly. Discussing skin care or waxing is appropriate with a makeup client. Go over the client questionnaire, making sure to ask the following questions: • Do you wear contacts or have skin sensitivities? • What type of look would you like to achieve? • What makeup products do you normally wear? • What are your typical clothing colors? • Are you going to a special occasion or event?			
2. Wash your hands.			
3. Drape the client and use a headband or hair clip to keep their hair out of their face.			
4. Cleanser—After washing your hands, cleanse the face if the client is wearing makeup or if the skin is oily.			
5. Toner—Use a cotton pad to apply toner to help remove any traces of makeup and restore the pH balance of the skin.			
6. Moisturizer—Apply a small amount of moisturizer to prepare the skin for makeup. Apply a primer if applicable.			
7. Lip conditioner—Use a new, single-use spatula to remove the product from the container. Apply with a disposable or disinfected brush. To give it more time to soak in and moisturize, put on the lip conditioner when starting the makeup application. Note: If lips are chapped, have clients rub off the dry skin with a wet washcloth, esthetic wipes, or a lip scrub before starting the service. Tissue or paper towels are drying and leave lint on the lips so are not recommended for this.			

8. Concealer—Use a spatula to remove the product from the container. Choose a color similar to the foundation and the same color as the skin.			
9. Match the surrounding skin closely in areas where you wish to cover darkness (under the eyes, over blemishes, over red or dark-colored splotches). You can use a concealer a shade lighter for highlighting. Apply with a brush or sponge, using short strokes. Note: Always use creams and liquids before applying powders for ease of blending. If you are using a powder concealer or contour powder, apply these after the foundation.			
10. Foundation—Select a few colors you wish to work with to blend and match the skin. Use a spatula to retrieve the product from the container, placing the product on a palette or directly on a disposable sponge. Apply to the jawline to check for a match with the skin.			
11. Cover the skin with a thin layer of product using even strokes. Blend along the jaw and edges of the face. Blend downward in the direction of the growth of facial hair and downward as well around the hairline. Pat gently around the eyes.			
12. Highlighter—Use a spatula to remove the product from the container. Apply a lighter color than the client's skin tone to accentuate and bring out features along the brow bone, temples, chin, or above the cheekbones. Blend well with a brush or sponge.			
13. Contouring—Use a spatula to get the product out of the container. Using a small amount, apply a darker shade under the cheekbones and to other features you want to appear smaller. Blend well.			
14. Powder—Pour a little powder on a clean palette or tissue to avoid cross-contamination.			
15. Apply to the brush and tap off excess powder onto the tissue. Use a powder brush and sweep all over the face to set the foundation.			
16. Eyebrows—Use a shade that is close to the hair color, or a shade the client likes. Brace your hand just above the brow and apply color by using short strokes with a pencil or eyeshadow with a brush.			
17. Smudge with a brush or a makeup sponge, going in the direction opposite to the hair growth to blend. Then smooth brows back into place with a brow brush.			

18. **Eyeshadow** Light—Choose a light base color and apply all over the eyelid, from the lash line up to the brow. Stop color at the outside corner of the eye up to the outside corner of the brow. To steady your hand and avoid eye injury, gently rest the base of your hand against the cheek of your client. Sometimes a tissue is used under your hand. For the eye, brace your hand just above the brow.			
19. Dark—Apply a darker shade to the crease: partially on top of the crease and partially underneath the crease. First tap the excess powder off the brush. Never blow on brushes. Apply the most color from the outside corner of the eye into the crease area above the inside of the iris.			
20. This dark color covers three-quarters of the way above the outside part of the eye. Blend the color. Optional: Apply the eyeliner before applying the dark shadow color.			
21. Choose an eyeliner—Sharpen the liner before and after use. Shadow as wet liner can also be used for liner and applied with a single-use or clean brush. Eyeshadow can be applied as liner with a thin brush dipped in water. Dry shadow can also be applied with a thin, firm brush for a more natural look. Make sure the liner is not too rough or so dry that it drags on the eye. Liquid liners require applicators that are disposable or that can be disinfected. Each dip into the liquid will require a new applicator.			
22. Apply eyeliner—Have the client shut their eyes when you apply the liner on top of the eyelids next to the lashes.			
23. Have the client look up and away as you apply the lower liner under the eyes. Apply the liner underneath the lower lashes.			
24. Complete the eyeliner and blend—Bring the liner three-quarters of the way from the outside edge of the eye in toward the center of the eye, ending softly at the inside of the iris. Blend so that the color tapers off. Bringing the liner in closer to the nose can make the eyes appear closer together. Lining only the outside corner makes the eyes appear farther apart. Make sure the line does not abruptly stop. Blend the liner with a firm, small liner brush.			
25. Mascara—Dip the disposable wand then wipe off excess product. Note: Some artists prefer to do the lower lashes first to avoid mascara touching the tops of the eye area when the client looks up for the lower application.			

26. Apply to lower lashes—Have the client put their chin down while looking up at the ceiling with their eyes to apply mascara to the bottom lashes. Be sure to brace the hand lightly on the face for more control. Comb and separate before the mascara dries.			
27. Apply to upper lashes—Wipe excess product off the wand. Have the client look down and focus on a fixed point to apply mascara to the upper lashes, brushing from the base to the tip. Be sure to brace the hand lightly on the face for more control. Use a lash comb before the product dries and before the client looks in a different direction to avoid smudging. Note: Use a cotton-tipped swab or small stiff brush with a little foundation or powder on it to fix or erase smudges. Optional: Curl the lashes before applying mascara. Hold the curler on the base of the lashes without pulling and release the curler before moving it away from the lashes.			
28. Blush—The order in which you apply blush is a personal choice. (Note: If you are using a cream blush, apply this before applying powders.) Tap off the excess powder from the brush. Apply blush just below the cheekbones, blending back and forth along the cheekbone. For optimum results, the color should stop below the temple and should not go lower than the nose. The blush domain area is no closer to the nostrils than the center of the pupil and no closer to the jawbone than an imaginary line from the tip of the nose to the middle of the ear. And blush should blend to the hairline, but not into it. A more horizontal application of blush will tend to widen the face, whereas a more vertical application will make it look narrower. Following the cheekbones usually works best.			
29. Optional: lip conditioner—This step applies if lips are dry or you did not already apply lip moisturizer. Use a spatula to get the product out of the container. Use a disposable brush to apply. Put on a lip moisturizer so it can soak in and moisturize before you start applying the liner. Note: Some artists use a primer or foundation on the lips under the lip color to help keep it on.			
30. Lip liner—Sharpen the liner. Have the client smile and stretch their lips. Brace at the corner of the mouth. With the lips pulled tight, the liner and lipstick brush glide on more smoothly. Line the outer edges of the lips first with small firm strokes; then fill in and use the liner as a lipstick. This keeps the lipstick and color on longer.			

31. Lipstick—Use a spatula to get the product out of the container. Have the client select a color from among two or three choices. Apply the lipstick evenly with a lip brush. Rest your ring finger near the client's chin to steady your hand. Ask the client to relax their lips and part them slightly. Brush on the lip color. Then ask the client to smile slightly so that you can smooth the lip color into any small crevices.			
32. Blot the lips with tissue to remove excess product and set the lip color. Finish with gloss if desired.			
33. Show the client the finished application—Remove the cape and hair clips so they can see the finished look. Discuss the colors and any product needs they may have.			
Post-Service			
Complete Procedures 7–2 and 8–9: Post-Service Procedures.			

PROCEDURE 12–2: APPLYING ARTIFICIAL LASHES

Evaluate your practical skills.

CRITERIA	COMPETENT	NEEDS WORK	IMPROVEMENT PLAN
Preparation			
Perform Procedures 7–1 and 8–1: Pre-Service Procedures.			
Discuss with the client the desired length of the lashes and the effect they hope to achieve.			
Wash your hands and put on gloves.			
Place the client in the makeup chair with their head at a comfortable working height. The client's face should be well and evenly lit; avoid shining the light directly into the eyes. Work from behind or to the side of the client. Avoid working directly in front of the client whenever possible.			
If the client wears contact lenses, she must remove them before starting the procedure.			
If the client is only having artificial lashes applied and you have not already done so, remove mascara so that the lash adhesive will adhere properly. Work carefully and gently. Follow the manufacturer's instructions carefully.			

Procedure			
1. Brush the client's eyelashes to make sure they are clean and free of foreign matter, such as mascara particles.			
2. If the client's lashes are straight, they can be curled with an eyelash curler before you apply the artificial lashes.			
3. Carefully remove the eyelash band from the package. Tweezers work well for this.			
4. Start with the upper lash. Hold this up to the eye to measure the length. Use your fingers to bend the lash into a horseshoe shape to make it more flexible so it fits the contour of the eyelid. If the band lash is too long to fit the curve of the upper eyelid, trim the outside edge.			
5. Feather straight band lashes to make uneven lengths on the end ("w" shapes) by nipping into them with the points of your scissors if desired. This creates a more natural look.			
6. Using a disposable brush or rounded end of a toothpick, apply a thin strip of lash adhesive to the base of the false lashes and allow a few seconds for it to set.			
7. Apply the lashes For strip lashes—Apply the lashes by holding the ends with the fingers or tweezers. Start with the shorter part of the lash and place it on the natural lashes at the inner corner of the eye, toward the nose. Note: You may wish to apply eyeliner before the lash is applied if it will not affect the false lash adhesion.			
8. Position the rest of the artificial lash as close to the client's own lash as possible, not on the skin. Make sure there is not an excess of glue and that the client can open their eyes once applied. Remove any excess glue and reposition the lashes as necessary.			
9. For individual lashes—Using tweezers, apply one at a time until you have five or six lashes that are evenly spaced across the lash line.			
10. Use longer lashes on the outer edges of the eye, medium length in the middle, and short on the inside by the nose. Cut lash lengths as needed.			
11. Use the rounded end of a lash liner brush, or tweezers, to press the lash on without adhering the brush or tweezers to the glue. Be very careful and gentle when applying the lashes. Remove any excess glue and rebrush or reposition lashes as necessary.			

12. An additional liquid liner may be used to finish the look if it does not affect the false lash adhesion. Adding a coat of mascara can help false lashes adhere to natural lashes.			
13. Optional: Apply the lower lash, if desired. Trim the lash as necessary. Scissors should not be used near the client's eyelashes as you might accidentally cut their natural lashes. Always cut the lashes away from the client. Once cut, place the lashes near the eye to check the size. If additional cutting is required, bring them down away from the client's eyes. When ready, apply adhesive in the same way you did for the upper lash. Place the lash on top of or beneath the client's lower lash. Place the shorter lash toward the center of the eye and the longer lash toward the outer part.			
14. Check the finished application and make sure the client is comfortable with the lashes. Remind the client to take special care with artificial lashes when swimming, bathing, and cleansing the face. Water, oil, or cleansing products will loosen artificial lashes. Band lash applications last one day and are meant to be removed nightly.			
Post-Service			
Complete Procedures 7–2 and 8–9: Post-Service Procedures.			

PROCEDURE 12–3: TINTING LASHES AND BROWS

Evaluate your practical skills.

CRITERIA	COMPETENT	NEEDS WORK	IMPROVEMENT PLAN
Preparation			
Perform Procedures 7–1 and 8–1: Pre-Service Procedures.			
Procedure			
1. Wash hands and put on gloves.			
2. Gather and set out supplies.			
3. Wet cotton pads and cotton swabs.			
4. Conduct the client consultation, and have the client sign the release form. Drape the client with a headband and towel around the neck.			
5. Cleanse the brow and/or lash area. All makeup must be removed and the area clean and dry before applying tint.			
6. Brush brows into place.			

7. Apply protective cream with a cotton swab directly next to the area where you are tinting to protect the skin, covering the area where you do not want the tint. Do not touch the hairs with cream because this interferes with the color. Apply cream around the brow area.			
8. Apply cream on the skin below the eye and above the lashes, just next to the lash line.			
9. Apply pads for lash tinting—Apply pads under the eyes and over the cream to keep tint from bleeding onto the skin. Use the paper sheaths in the tint kit. You may have to cut or adjust pad shapes to fit under the eyes. Pads should be under the lashes as close to the eye as possible without holding or interfering with the lower lashes. To make cotton pads—Wet the pads and squeeze out excess water, tearing them so they are half as thick. Then fold in half to make half-moon-shaped pads.			
10. Adjust the pads—Have the client close their eyes, and adjust the pad so it sits next to the eye, not bunched up too close to the eye. If the pad is too close or too wet, tint may wick into the eye and onto the skin.			
11. Prepare your timer according to the manufacturer's directions and have wet pads and cotton swabs ready to use for rinsing. Note: You can start with the lashes and do the brows while the lash tint is processing. Generally, tint can sit on the lashes longer than the brows if you are going for a natural brow look.			
12. Prepare the tint— Place the amount of product you need into a cup-shaped palette. The brow tint can be diluted with water in a 1:1 ratio in a mixing cup to lighten the color.			
13. Some tint kits have only one bottle and combine the tint and developer into one application. If your kit requires the addition of developer to the tint be sure to add it at this time and mix well.			
14. Apply the lash tint—For the lashes, brush the product from the base of the lashes to the ends. Do not double-dip—use a new applicator each time to reapply. Note: Some manufacturers may suggest a second layer of protective sheaths that may be fitted over the tinted lashes at this time.			
15. Apply the brow tint—For the brows, apply the color from the inside to the outside edge. Do not double-dip—use a new applicator each time to reapply and work across the brows. Caution: Brows can absorb color quickly, so be ready to remove it right away to avoid excess color.			

16. Begin the timer and leave on for three minutes or as directed. If your kit requires the application of developer in a separate step, use a new applicator to carefully apply the developer (bottle #2 for some kits) for one minute or as directed.			
17. Rinse each area with water at least three times with wet cotton swabs and cotton pads without dripping water into the eyes. Have an emergency eyewash kit available in case any product gets into the client's eye.			
18. Remove the protective pads and continue to rinse the area thoroughly.			
19. Ask the client if they feel any discomfort and have them flush the eyes with water at the sink if necessary. It is common for the eyes to feel a little grainy after tinting, so rinsing is a good idea. Show the application to the client.			
Post-Service			
Complete Procedures 7–2 and 8–9: Post-Service Procedures.			

CHAPTER 13
ADVANCED TOPICS AND TREATMENTS

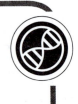

EXPLAIN ADVANCED SKIN CARE TOPICS AND TREATMENTS FOR LICENSED, TRAINED ESTHETICIANS

SHORT ANSWER

1. Why should estheticians study advanced topics and treatments?

_____

_____

_____

_____

_____

_____

_____

_____

DESCRIBE CHEMICAL EXFOLIATION AND PEELS

SHORT ANSWER

2. What is chemical exfoliation and how could this treatment help a client with hyperpigmentation?

_____

_____

_____

_____

_____

_____

_____

_____

Acid, Alkaline, and pH Relationships

FILL IN THE BLANK

3. _____ are added to products to help make them less irritating.

4. _____ have a pH of 0 to 6.

5. A pH less than _____ is not recommended for peels.

6. Ingredients added to products to help make them less irritating are called _____.

7. The cell turnover rate, or _____, is the rate of cell mitosis and migration from the dermis to the top of the epidermis.

SHORT ANSWER

8. List the six factors that can influence aging of the skin.

- _____
- _____
- _____
- _____
- _____
- _____

Light, Medium, and Deep Peels—What Is the Difference?

FILL IN THE BLANK

9. A light peel is administered by a(n) _____. Medium and deep peels are administered by a(n) _____.

10. Removing cells from the stratum corneum is known as _____ or _____.

SHORT ANSWER

11. How are light peels different from medium and deep peels?

_____

_____

_____

_____

_____

_____

_____

_____

_____

_____

General Effects of Chemical Exfoliation and Peels

SHORT ANSWER

12. List the beneficial effects of peels and chemical exfoliations.

- _____
- _____
- _____
- _____
- _____
- _____

General Contraindications to and Precautions for Chemical Exfoliation and Peels

SHORT ANSWER

13. What advice should you give your client after a chemical exfoliation and peel?

_____
_____
_____
_____
_____

IDENTIFY HOW TO SAFELY AND EFFECTIVELY USE CHEMICAL EXFOLIATION AND PEELS

SHORT ANSWER

14. List the four types of peels and chemical exfoliations.

- _____
- _____
- _____
- _____

What Is an Enzyme Peel?

FILL IN THE BLANK

15. An enzyme peel may also be referred to as a(n) enzyme _____ or enzyme _____.

16. Enzymes are _____ in nature and work to _____ the keratin (protein) in dead skin cells on the surface of the skin.

SHORT ANSWER

17. When is an enzyme peel a good choice for your client?

_____

_____

_____

_____

_____

18. List the factors you should consider before providing your client with an enzyme peel.

_____

_____

_____

_____

_____

_____

_____

_____

_____

_____

_____

TRUE OR FALSE

19. For the following statements discussing contraindications and best practices, circle *T* if true or *F* if false.

T   F   Eyewear is not required when applying an enzyme peel.

T   F   Some areas of the face may process sooner than others and require spot removal.

T   F   Be prepared to remove the peel just prior to the end point.

T   F   The application of moisturizer and a product containing SPF is not required after an enzyme peel.

T   F   Before the application process, be sure to cleanse and tone the skin.

PERFORM AN ENZYME MASK TREATMENT

FILL IN THE BLANK

20. Place the following steps of an enzyme mask treatment in the correct order on the blanks below. Number them from 1 to start.

_____ Apply a cleanser to remove makeup.

_____ Remove the mask using 4" × 4" moistened esthetics wipes or chosen material.

_____ Properly drape the client and wash your hands.

_____ Remove the cleanser residue using 2" × 2" gauze pads or cotton rounds moistened with toner.

_____ Discuss your observations and any recommendations with the client.

_____ Apply the enzyme mask.

_____ Apply moisturizer and sun protection.

_____ Perform a visual analysis of the skin.

_____ Perform proper post-service.

_____ Apply goggles to your client and yourself to protect the eyes from any irritants.

_____ Process the mask according to the manufacturer's instructions.

_____ Apply toner to the skin to remove mask residue.

_____ Remove your gloves and wash your hands.

What is an AHA or a BHA Peel?

FILL IN THE BLANK

21. AHA is an acronym for _____.

22. AHAs penetrate the _____ and aid in dissolving _____ to keep skin cells _____.

23. _____ acid is the strongest AHA and can penetrate the epidermis because it has the smallest molecular size.

24. BHAs have _____ and _____ properties.

25. BHAs include _____ which is derived from sweet birch, willow bark, and wintergreen.

26. For clients with oily skin and acne, it is often best to use a peel that contains _____.

MATCHING

27. Match the following AHAs with their sources:

apples	citrus fruit	milk
bitter almond	grapes	sugar cane

Lactic acid   _____

Mandelic acid   _____

Tartaric acid   _____

Glycolic acid   _____

Citric acid   _____

Malic acid   _____

SHORT ANSWER

28. How does a BHA differ from an AHA?

_____

_____

_____

_____

_____

29. With the help of the client's intake form, list all factors that you should consider before suggesting or providing an AHA or BHA peel to your client.

_____

_____

_____

_____

_____

_____

_____

_____

_____

_____

30. List the factors that you should discuss with your client before providing an AHA or BHA peel.

_____

_____

_____

_____

_____

_____

_____

_____

_____

_____

_____

_____

_____

_____

_____

FILL IN THE BLANK

31. Before scheduling treatments, it is important to note the condition of the skin on the _____.

32. When performing the peel consultation and throughout the process, always keep in mind the manufacturer's _____.

33. _____ must be worn at all times by the client and the esthetician.

34. As an additional precaution, you may apply _____ to the corners of the eyes, the mouth, and around the nostril area.

35. Chemical exfoliation and other exfoliation procedures should be used with extreme caution during the _____ due to the high risk of sun exposure.

36. A _____ may be used during the BHA application to view the accuracy and evenness of the peel application.

37. Identify the proper order in the general peel application process by placing a number beside each step below.

_____ Apply moisturizer.

_____ Process the peel.

_____ Rinse the peel.

_____ Apply SPF product.

_____ Cleanse.

_____ Apply the peel.

_____ Neutralize the peel.

_____ Tone.

PERFORM A LIGHT GLYCOLIC PEEL

FILL IN THE BLANK

38. Place the following steps of a light glycolic peel in the correct order on the blanks below. Number them from 1 to start.

_____ Neutralize the peel.

_____ Carefully analyze the client's skin with the magnifying lamp.

_____ Apply moisturizer and sun protection liberally.

_____ Apply a cleanser, massage in circular motions, then remove.

_____ Complete the proper pre-service.

_____ Remove the peel.

_____ Apply the peel.

_____ Wash your hands and put on gloves.

_____ Use toner to remove residue.

_____ Apply a protective ointment around the eyes, corners of the nose, and on the lips.

_____ Cleanse and analyze the skin.

_____ Apply protective eyewear to your client and yourself.

_____ Process the peel.

_____ Remove your gloves and wash your hands.

_____ Discuss your observations and any recommendations with the client.

What Is a Jessner's or a TCA Peel?

39. A Jessner's peel is a mixture of _____ , _____ , _____ ,
    and _____ .

40. TCA is an acronym for _____ .

41. Due to _____ , both Jessner's and TCA peels will cause flaking and peeling.

SHORT ANSWER

42. What is a Jessner's or TCA peel and what are the benefits of each?

_____

_____

_____

_____

_____

43. With the help of the client's intake form, list all factors that you should consider before suggesting or
    providing a Jessner's or TCA peel to your client.

_____

_____

_____

_____

_____

_____

_____

_____

_____

44. List the factors that you should discuss with your client prior to providing a Jessner's or TCA
    peel.

_____

_____

_____

_____

_____

_____

_____

_____

_____

_____

_____

_____

_____

_____

_____

FILL IN THE BLANK

45. Pretreatment and home care guidelines may include products that address aging or sun damage such as _____ or _____ .

46. For clients with oily and acneic skin, you may add in products such as an _____ and _____ serum.

47. The Jessner's solution is usually applied in _____ , according to the manufacturer's directions.

48. An example of a treatment series is _____ TCA peels administered _____ every three to four weeks, then moving to maintenance with lower-dose peels such as a 30 percent AHA once a month.

49. Identify the proper order in the Jessner's and TCA peel application process by placing a number beside each step below.

_____ Apply moisturizer.

_____ Process the peel.

_____ Rinse the peel (if directed).

_____ Apply SPF product.

_____ Cleanse.

_____ Apply the peel.

_____ Neutralize the peel.

_____ Tone.

What Is a Designer Peel?

SHORT ANSWER

50. What differentiates a designer peel from other peels?

_____

_____

_____

_____

_____

DISCUSS THE BENEFITS OF MICRODERMABRASION BY TYPE OF DEVICE

FILL IN THE BLANK

51. Microdermabrasion is a machine-based exfoliation treatment that uses a _____ or _____ to gently polish dead skin cells from the skin's surface.

Crystal Microdermabrasion

FILL IN THE BLANK

52. Using a hand piece, the crystal microdermabrasion procedure sprays high-grade microcrystals composed of _____, _____, or a similar abrasive material across the skin's surface.

53. A _____ should be worn at all times due to the crystal residue that is both messy and a respiratory hazard.

54. _____ is gentler on the skin and does not require the use of a machine.

Crystal-Free Microdermabrasion

SHORT ANSWER

55. Why is crystal-free microdermabrasion becoming more popular than crystal microdermabrasion?

_____

_____

_____

_____

_____

Hydradermabrasion (Wet Dermabrasion)

FILL IN THE BLANK

56. Hydradermabrasion combines _____ and _____ exfoliation with serum penetration and _____ via a machine similar to the closed loop system of a crystal microdermabrasion machine.

57. A hand piece is used with _____ and an abrasive tip to provide a deep cleansing, extraction, and exfoliation action.

SHORT ANSWER

58. What are the benefits of providing a hydradermabrasion treatment?

_____

_____

_____

_____

_____

Timing and Technique

FILL IN THE BLANK

59. Microdermabrasion treatments are quick _____ services that can be offered alone or as part of a facial as well as part of an advanced treatment such as LED.

60. List at least three key factors to a successful microdermabrasion technique.

- _____

- _____

- _____

- _____

- _____

61. The end point for a microdermabrasion treatment is the presence of _____.

62. Use of the microdermabrasion machine requires _____ and _____ and should be used by licensed, trained skin care professionals only.

SHORT ANSWER

63. What are the differences between microdermabrasion and an AHA peel, and which is preferred for a client looking to stimulate their skin's turnover rate?

_____

_____

_____

_____

_____

_____

_____

_____

SHORT ANSWER

64. List five conditions that may diminish with microdermabrasion.

- _____

- _____

- _____

- _____

- _____

65. With the help of the client's intake form, list all factors that you should consider before suggesting or providing microdermabrasion to your client.

_____

_____

_____

_____

_____

_____

_____

_____

_____

_____

_____

_____

_____

_____

_____

_____

_____

FILL IN THE BLANK

66. End the treatment when the skin shows signs of _____ or _____ .

67. _____ and _____ must wear protective eyewear to avoid eye damage. _____ must wear masks to avoid breathing in crystals.

68. Avoid getting crystals in the client's _____, _____, or _____.

69. Improper use of microdermabrasion can lead to sensitivity, _____, and _____ .

70. A treatment plan series can consist of _____ to _____ microdermabrasion treatments administered once a week over _____ to _____ weeks.

TRUE OR FALSE

71. For the following statements, circle *T* if true or *F* if false.

    T F   During the maintenance phase, you maintain the results by administering a daily maintenance microdermabrasion treatment.

    T F   Photo documentation before and after treatments and is a good business practice for your personal records and beneficial documentation of the client's progress.

    T F   A constant, even flow of crystals will give a smooth and effective treatment.

    T F   A mask and gloves are not required when cleaning up the crystals.

EXPLAIN THE BENEFITS OF LASER TECHNOLOGY

FILL IN THE BLANK

72. Lasers are medical devices used for _____ and _____.

73. Laser is an acronym that stands for _____.

74. Lasers are high-powered devices that use intense pulses of _____ and a single _____ at one time.

75. Lasers are designed to focus all of the light power with the same color, traveling to a specific depth, in one _____ .

76. Intense pulsed light (IPL) has multiple colors, _____, and _____ and the light may be _____.

77. The equipment you use in light therapy is selected based on the _____ and _____ you are treating.

78. Different _____ affect different components of the skin.

When to Use and Effects of Laser Technology

FILL IN THE BLANK

79. All lasers and light therapy methods use selective _____.

80. Lasers emit light waves of the same _____.

81. Nonlaser photo devices, such as IPL, use a _____ of different wavelengths.

82. A laser produces _____ light.

SHORT ANSWER

83. Explain the benefits of using laser technology.

_____

_____

_____

_____

_____

EXPLAIN THE BENEFITS AND TYPES OF LIGHT THERAPY

FILL IN THE BLANK

84. Light therapy is the application of light rays to the skin for the treatment of _____,
_____ , _____ , or _____

85. The range of wavelengths used in light therapy are _____ , _____ , and
_____ .

What Is Infrared Light and When Do You Use It?

SHORT ANSWER

86. What is infrared light and what are the potential benefits for your client?

_____

_____

_____

_____

_____

_____

_____

_____

_____

_____

_____

What Is IPL and When Do You Use It?

FILL IN THE BLANK

87. IPL devices use pulses of multiple wavelengths to reduce _____ , _____
_____ , and rejuvenate the skin.

88. Intense pulse light emits light absorbed by _____ , _____ , and hair
follicles.

89. A nonablative treatment that utilizes light therapy for the extrinsic and intrinsic signs of again is
known as _____ .

What Are the Effects of IPL?

SHORT ANSWER

90. List five conditions that can be treated with an IPL device.

_____

- _____
- _____
- _____
- _____
- _____

What LED Is and When to Use It

FILL IN THE BLANK

91. LED is the acronym for _____ .

92. An LED treatment does not use heat; therefore, it is _____ .

93. _____ , also known as LED technology, works on the premise of nonablative cellular stimulation.

94. An LED treatment differs from a laser as there is no risk of _____ to your client.

SHORT ANSWER

95. List five of the many benefits your client may experience from an LED treatment.

Effects of an LED Treatment

MATCHING

96. Match the benefit to the color of the LED light.

a. red light	c. green light
b. yellow light	d. blue light

_____ improves lymphatic flow

_____ improves acne

_____ lessens hyperpigmentation

_____ reduces redness

_____ boosts collagen and elastin production

_____ calms and soothes

_____ reduces inflammation

_____ reduces bacteria

_____ detoxifies and increases circulation

_____ stimulates wound healing

_____ may be used with medications for precancerous lesions in a medical setting only

_____ increases cellular processes

Contraindications and Best Practices for LED

SHORT ANSWER

97. List the contraindications that could prevent your client from receiving an LED treatment.

- _____

- _____

- _____

- _____

- _____

- _____

- _____

- _____

- _____

- _____

- _____

Safety and Maintenance for LED Machines

FILL IN THE BLANK

98. After every treatment, be sure to _____ the machines and protective eyewear.

DISCUSS MICROCURRENT TREATMENTS

FILL IN THE BLANK

99. Microcurrent is also known as _____.

100. Microcurrent devices mimic the way the _____ relays messages to the muscles.

101. The electrical current is regulated according to the skin's _____.

102. For visible results, treatments are given once a week for at least _____ sessions and every _____ weeks.

103. Microcurrent is used to relax muscles, and strengthen and tone the muscles by stimulating _____ and contractions of the muscles.

When to Use Microcurrent

SHORT ANSWER

104. List some of the benefits of using microcurrent.

- _____
_____

- _____
_____

- _____
_____

Effects of Microcurrent

FILL IN THE BLANK

105. Microcurrent is used primarily to _____ and _____ facial muscles.

106. Microcurrent is considered a _____ form of exercise.

107. It has the ability to firm muscles, boost cellular activity, and improve blood and lymph _____.

Contraindications and Precautions for Microcurrent

FILL IN THE BLANK

108. List the contraindications that could prevent the use of microcurrent.

- _____

- _____

- _____

- _____

- _____

- _____

- _____

- _____

- _____

- _____

Best Practices and Safety Considerations for Microcurrent

FILL IN THE BLANK

109. The microcurrent treatment requires proper positioning and an understanding of muscle _____, _____, and _____ .

Safety and Maintenance of Microcurrent

FILL IN THE BLANK

110. Be sure to maintain your machines in accordance with the manufacturer's instructions and always disinfect the _____ and _____ after each use.

DISCUSS ULTRASOUND

FILL IN THE BLANK

111. Ultrasound and _____ are synonymous terms referring to a frequency that is above the range of sound audible to the human ear.

112. Results-oriented treatments are achieved by using noninvasive _____ waves.

113. Ultrasonic equipment is based on _____ mechanical oscillations produced by a metal spatula-like tool.

When to Use and Effects of Ultrasound Technology

FILL IN THE BLANK

114. Ultrasound penetrates deeply to _____ tissue, _____ blood flow, and promote _____ .

115. For ultrasound, the _____ the frequency, the greater the penetration; conversely, a _____ frequency has less penetration.

116. Ultrasound can affect _____ through the heat manipulation of the tissue and lymphatic movements performed with the device.

117. Heat damage from ultrasound and other modalities stimulates _____ production.

118. The process of ultrasound sending waves through the skin to assist in product penetration is called _____ .

Contraindications and Precautions for Ultrasound Technology

SHORT ANSWER

119. List six contraindications for ultrasound.

- _____
- _____
- _____
- _____
- _____
- _____

Safety and Maintenance for Ultrasound Machines

FILL IN THE BLANK

120. Ultrasound machines should be maintained according to the manufacturer's instructions and disinfected _____ .

Microneedling or Dermal Rolling

SHORT ANSWER

121. Explain the differences between microneedling (dermal rolling) and Nano infusion.

_____

_____

_____

_____

_____

_____

_____

_____

_____

DESCRIBE SPA BODY TREATMENTS

MATCHING

122. Match the body treatment with its description below.

a. ayurvedic	b. balneotherapy	c. body masks	d. body scrubs
e. body wraps	f. endermology	g. energy practices	h. foot reflexology
i. hydrotherapy	j. reiki	k. stone massage	l. sunless tanning

_____ Japanese technique for stress reduction and relaxation that also promotes healing

_____ include energy and chakra balancing

_____ alternative to tanning that includes product application by spray or manually

_____ treatment of physical ailments using therapeutic water baths

_____ treatments where product is applied on the body and then covered or wrapped up

_____ treatment that uses water in its three forms

_____ uses friction to exfoliate and hydrate, increase circulation, and nourish skin using a combination of ingredients

_____ technique of using hot stones and cold stones in massage or other treatments

_____ treatment based on the three doshas that include shirodhara, massage, and facials

_____ treatment that helps stimulate the reduction of adipose tissue by vacuum massage

_____ technique of applying pressure to the feet based on a system of zones and areas that directly correspond to the anatomy of the body

_____ treatment that remineralizes and detoxifies the body using primarily clay, mud, or seaweed mixtures

DISCUSS COMMON TREATMENTS USED TO ADDRESS CELLULITE

SHORT ANSWER

123. What are some effective ways to treat cellulite?

_____

_____

_____

_____

_____

EXPLAIN THE BENEFITS OF MANUAL LYMPH DRAINAGE

FILL IN THE BLANK

124. Manual lymph drainage stimulates _____ to flow through the lymphatic vessels.

When to Use Manual Lymph Drainage and Effects of This Modality

FILL IN THE BLANK

125. Manual lymph drainage uses massage to help cleanse and _____ the body.

126. Congestion, water, and waste in the lymphatic vessels create _____ in the tissue.

127. When used after surgery, it can expedite _____ and enhance cell metabolism.

DISCUSS THE FIELD OF MEDICAL ESTHETICS

SHORT ANSWER

128. What is the role of a clinical esthetician in a medical esthetics setting and what types of treatments might one provide to their clients?

_____

_____

_____

_____

_____

FILL IN THE BLANK

129. _____ are medical clinics and spas combined in one location and offer both esthetic and medical services.

130. The most popular medical spa services are:

- _____

- _____

- _____

- _____

- _____

- _____

131. Pre-operative care focuses on _____ the skin for the procedure.

132. Getting the skin in its optimum state and as healthy as possible makes the surgery less _____ on the tissue and _____ recovery time.

133. Post-op care includes providing skin care for rapid wound healing and the avoidance of _____ .

134. Massage, hydration, protection, and _____ are often part of post-op care.

135. _____ procedures do not remove tissue.

MATCHING

136. Match the term with its description. The terms will be used more than once.

a. Botox®	b. dermal fillers

_____ fills lines, wrinkles, and other facial imperfections

_____ neuromuscular-blocking serum

_____ causes paralysis or diminished movement by blocking neurotransmitters

_____ collagen treatment may be made of a bovine derivative

_____ may be made from synthetic sources such as silicone and hyaluronic acids

_____ relaxes tissues and diminishes lines

_____ glabella is the most common injected site

FILL IN THE BLANK

137. A forehead lift is also called a _____ .

138. _____ minimizes varicose veins (dilated blood vessels) and other varicosities by injecting chemical agents into the affected areas.

WORD REVIEW

FILL IN THE BLANK

139. Provide the correct vocabulary term for each.

The _____ is the rate of cell mitosis and migration from the dermis to the top of the epidermis.

A _____ is categorized as a stronger superficial peel and utilizes a mixture of salicylic acid, resorcinol, lactic acid, and ethanol.

_____ is a machine-based exfoliation treatment that uses a crystal spray or diamond tips to gently polish dead skin cells from the skin's surface.

_____ are high-powered medical devices that use intense pulses of electromagnetic radiation and a single wavelength at one time for hair removal and skin treatments.

_____ use pulses of multiple wavelengths (versus single in lasers) to reduce pigmentation, remove surface capillaries, and rejuvenate the skin.

A _____, is a nonthermal device used to reduce acne, increase skin circulation, and improve the collagen content in the skin.

A _____ is a color component within the skin such as blood or melanin.

_____ in LED therapy increases cellular processes, boosts collagen and elastin production, and stimulates wound healing.

_____ in LED therapy reduces inflammation, improves lymphatic flow, detoxifies and increases circulation.

_____ in LED therapy lessens hyperpigmentation, reduces redness, and calms and soothes.

_____ in LED therapy improves acne and reduces bacteria and may be used with medications on precancerous lesions.

_____, or wave therapy, devices mimic the way the brain relays messages to the muscles which can be used to treat many conditions, such as Bell's palsy and stroke paralysis.

_____ equipment is based on high-frequency mechanical oscillations produced by a metal spatula- like tool.

_____ stimulates tissue, increases blood flow, and promotes oxygenation and can be used for product penetration and cellulite reduction by helping to cleanse and exfoliate the skin by removing dead skin cells.

_____ or dermal rolling is a cosmetic and medical rolling form of collagen induction therapy (CIT).

_____ are treatments where product is applied on the body and then covered or wrapped up.

_____ use friction to exfoliate and hydrate, increase circulation, and nourish skin using a combination of ingredients such as ground nuts, apricot kernels, cornmeal, jojoba beads, honey, salt, or sugar combined with oil or lotion.

_____ remineralize and detoxify the body using primarily clay, mud, or seaweed mixtures.

_____ is spa treatment that uses water in its three forms.

_____ is the treatment of physical ailments using therapeutic water baths.

_____ is the technique of using hot stones and cold stones in massage or other treatments.

_____ is the technique of applying pressure to the feet based on a system of zones and areas on the feet that directly correspond to the anatomy of the body.

_____ concepts are based on three doshas and include Shirodhara, massage, and facials using ancient Indian concepts and ingredients suited to the three body/mind types: pitta, kapha, and vatta.

_____ is a treatment for cellulite that helps stimulate the reduction of adipose tissue by a vacuum massage that combines a vigorous massage along with suction.

_____ is a Japanese technique for stress reduction and relaxation that also promotes healing.

_____ consists of fat cells and appears as dimpled or bumpy skin caused primarily by female hormones and genetics. Cellulite consists of fat cells.

_____ procedures do not remove tissue.

_____ are substances used in nonsurgical procedures to fill in or plump up areas of the skin.

_____ is a neuromuscular-blocking serum that paralyzes nerve cells on the muscle when this serum is injected into it.

_____ are used to fill lines, wrinkles, and other facial imperfections.

_____ is defined as that which restores a bodily function.

_____ , also known as esthetic surgery, is elective surgery for improving and altering the appearance.

A _____ is a facelift.

A _____ is an eye lift.

A _____ is performed inside the lower eyelid to remove bulging fat pads.

_____ is a nose surgery.

_____ is used to smooth wrinkles or lighten acne scars.

_____ is a strong exfoliation method that uses a mechanical brush to physically remove tissue down to the dermis.

_____ peels are deep peels used to address sun damage and wrinkles.

_____ peels are the strongest peels and can be toxic.

_____ is breast surgery that enlarges the breasts or reconstructs them.

_____ is the procedure that surgically removes pockets of fat.

_____ removes excessive fat deposits and loose skin from the abdomen to tuck and tighten the area.

DISCOVERIES AND ACCOMPLISHMENTS

In the space below, write notes about key concepts discussed in this chapter. Share at least five of your discoveries with two of the other students in your class and ask for feedback on your notes. Write five additional discoveries based on good ideas shared by your peers.

Discoveries:

_____

_____

_____

_____

_____

_____

_____

_____

_____

_____

_____

_____

List at least three things you have accomplished since your last entry that relate to your career goals.

Accomplishments:

_____

_____

_____

_____

_____

_____

_____

_____

_____

_____

_____

_____

EXAM REVIEW

MULTIPLE CHOICE

1. As a spa owner, it is important to encourage your staff to continue their education in advanced skin care topics because _____.

    a. advanced machine technology is always evolving

    b. if they don't, you could lower their salaries

    c. many techniques have remained the same for decades

    d. it will keep your spa up-to-date with legal regulation.

2. Which of these statements about LED light is true?

    a. LED light is used for skin rejuvenation.

    b. Different colors of LED light produce different effects on the skin.

    c. LED light can help improve acne.

    d. All of the answers are correct.

3. What is a TCA peel used for?

    a. lightening highly pigmented skin

    b. darkening lightly pigmented skin

    c. diminishing sun damage and wrinkles

    d. preventing collagen and elastin production

4. What happens to the cell renewal factor as you age?

    a. It improves.   c. It speeds up.

    b. It becomes more efficient.   d. It slows down.

5. What is a normal pH for skin?

    a. 0–2   c. 7–8

    b. 4.5–5.5   d. 9.5–10.15

6. What is true of open sores and suspicious lesions?

    a. They have no bearing on the choice to perform chemical exfoliation.

    b. They can be covered with gauze as you exfoliate the skin.

    c. They should never be mentioned on the client's intake form.

    d. These conditions always contraindicate chemical exfoliation.

7. What is **NOT** something that clients should be advised to avoid for at least 24 to 48 hours in advance of a chemical exfoliation procedure?

    a. showering   c. benzoyl peroxide applications

    b. sun exposure   d. waxing

8. A person with what condition would be a better candidate for microdermabrasion versus other forms of exfoliation?

    a. oily skin
    c. loose skin

    b. dry skin
    d. inability to tolerate acids

9. What treatment can have the effects of hyperpigmentation, hypopigmentation, and/or sensitivity if administered improperly?

    a. paraffin masks
    c. extraction

    b. clay masks
    d. microdermabrasion

10. A client wants to relax and detoxify her entire body. What would you recommend?

    a. a seaweed body wrap
    c. endermology

    b. microdermabrasion
    d. dermal fillers

11. You are recommending a microcurrent treatment to a client. Which of the following is **NOT** a result your client should expect?

    a. improved circulation
    c. cellulite reduction

    b. boosted cellular activity
    d. firm muscles

12. What are commonly used in balneotherapy body treatments?

    a. powerful water jets
    c. hot stones

    b. Dead Sea salts
    d. cold stones

13. What is **NOT** a benefit of body scrubs?

    a. reduced adipose tissue
    c. exfoliation

    b. increased circulation
    d. hydration

14. What **PRIMARILY** determines the effect of a body wrap?

    a. material used to wrap the client

    b. type of product used

    c. length of time the client is wrapped

    d. positioning of the client while wrapped

15. What is Botox®?

    a. highly acidic cream

    b. neuromuscular-blocking serum

    c. type of acne medication

    d. surgical procedure for removing fat from the abdomen

16. A client has an upcoming surgery. What procedure might the client undergo before and after the surgery to enhance cell metabolism?

    a. injectable fillers

    b. manual lymph drainage

    c. microdermabrasion

    d. light therapy

17. Which of the following is good advice for your clients after receiving a spa treatment?

    a. to lay down for the rest of the day and recharge her body

    b. to drink lots of water

    c. not to eat for several hours after treatment

    d. not to drive herself home

18. What does the aesthetician use to move congestion, water, and waste in the lymphatic vessels out of the body when performing MLD?

    a. massage

    b. microcurrent

    c. galvanic current

    d. reiki

19. What device mimics the body's natural electrical energy to re-educate and tone facial muscles?

    a. laser machine

    b. steamer

    c. microcurrent machine

    d. microdermabrasion machine

20. What is a form of mechanical exfoliation?

    a. mammoplasty

    b. microdermabrasion

    c. manual lymph drainage

    d. microcurrent

21. What type of treatment would be considered nonablative?

    a. a treatment that causes excessive skin friction

    b. a treatment that does not remove tissue

    c. a treatment that exfoliates

    d. a treatment that is injectable

22. What treatments employ the use of phenol (carbolic acid)?

    a. peels

    b. extractions

    c. exfoliations

    d. massages

23. Which of the following is **NOT** an option for treating cellulite?

    a. ultrasound

    b. exfoliation

    c. endermology

    d. Reiki

24. What is a rhytidectomy?

    a. tummy tuck

    b. breast enhancement

    c. face lift

    d. nose job

25. Which type of light is used for relaxation and the heating of muscles?

    a. infrared light

    b. UV light

    c. white light

    d. visible light

26. What condition does endermology treat?

    a. acne

    b. albinism

    c. sensitive skin

    d. cellulite

27. What is the technical term for an eye lift?

    a. rhinoplasty

    b. blepharoplasty

    c. oculoplasty

    d. hippoplasty

28. What is the term for spa treatments that use water?

    a. aqua therapy

    b. hydrotherapy

    c. liquid therapy

    d. immersion therapy

29. What purpose do injectable fillers serve?

    a. skin lightening

    b. stress relief

    c. skin darkening

    d. skin plumping

30. What is the term for the application of light rays to the skin for the treatment of wrinkles, capillaries, pigmentation, and hair removal?

    a. sclerotherapy

    b. endotherapy

    c. ultrasonic therapy

    d. light therapy

31. Which layer of the skin may be affected by a deep peel?

    a. dermal layer

    b. epidermis

    c. stratum corneum

    d. All of the answers are correct.

32. Which of the following treatments may increase collagen production during the wound healing process, but may not be permitted in some states?

    a. microneedling

    b. a medium peel

    c. a body wrap

    d. balneotherapy

33. What is **NOT** an ingredient of a Jessner's peel?

    a. citric acid

    b. lactic acid

    c. salicylic acid

    d. resorcinol

34. Which is true about crystal microdermabrasion?

    a. A mask is not needed during this treatment.

    b. Crystals are sprayed onto the skin.

    c. There is no need for additional clean up.

    d. Eyewear is not required.

35. Lasers are designed to _____.

    a. focus all the light-power with same color, traveling to a specific depth, in one direction

    b. have multiple colors, depths, and wavelengths

    c. have the same wavelength regardless of the component of the skin being treated

    d. use a low intensity electromagnetic radiation of multiple wavelengths

36. Ultrasound is known to _____.

    a. promote hair growth

    b. penetrate deeply

    c. be extremely abrasive

    d. keep dead skin cells intact

37. Which of the following should be encouraged to help avoid hyperpigmentation after exfoliation?

    a. a deep chemical peel

    b. rubbing the skin

    c. applying sunscreen daily

    d. applying a scrub

38. What should you suggest to your client to help achieve maximum results before, during, and even after receiving their treatment?

    a. avoid products containing AHAs or vitamin C

    b. avoid all cleansers

    c. follow a home care regimen

    d. schedule a peel for every day of the week

39. This treatment is noninvasive and uses a needle-free microneedling hand piece.

    a. Nano infusion

    b. sclerotherapy

    c. reflexology

    d. dermabrasion

40. This treatment uses a mechanical brush to physically remove tissue down to the dermis.

    a. dermabrasion

    b. enzyme mask

    c. laser therapy

    d. microneedling

PROCEDURE 13–1: PERFORM AN ENZYME MASK SERVICE

Evaluate your practical skills.

CRITERIA	COMPETENT	NEEDS WORK	IMPROVEMENT PLAN
Procedure			
1. Complete Procedure 7–1: Pre-Service including proper draping. Ensure the client is cleared for this service prior to proceeding. Discuss the expected outcome of this treatment with the client so they have realistic expectations of what the treatment can and cannot accomplish.			
2. Wash your hands and put on gloves.			
3. Perform a visual analysis of the skin to ensure the skin is intact and to ensure the treatment is not contraindicated. Complete Procedure 5–1: Skin Analysis.			
4. Apply a cleanser suitable to remove makeup with your gloved hands. Massage the cleanser to loosen makeup. Remove the cleanser.			
5. Using 2" x 2" gauze pads or cotton rounds moistened with toner, remove any residue.			
6. Apply goggles to your client and yourself to protect the eyes from any irritants.			
7. Using a disposable spatula or fan brush, apply the enzyme mask beginning at the forehead and moving to the temples, then to the right and left cheeks, chin, upper lip, and nose.			
8. Set a timer and process the mask according to the manufacturer's instructions. NOTE: Remove sooner if client cannot tolerate the treatment or if the peel has processed prior to the recommended minimal end time. Endpoint goal: very light erythema.			
9. Remove the mask using 4" x 4" moistened esthetics wipes or chosen material.			
10. Apply toner to the skin to remove residue.			
11. Apply moisturizer and sun protection.			
12. Remove your gloves and wash your hands.			
13. Discuss your observations and any recommendations with the client.			
14. Perform Procedure 7–2 and 8–9: Post-Service.			

PROCEDURE 13–2: PERFORM A BACK FACIAL WITH ENZYME MASK

Evaluate your practical skills.

CRITERIA	COMPETENT	NEEDS WORK	IMPROVEMENT PLAN
Procedure			
1. Complete Procedure 7–1: Pre-Service. Ensure the client is cleared for this service prior to proceeding.			
2. Cleanse and analyze the skin. Apply a cleanser suitable for the client's skin type with your gloved hands. Massage the cleanser in circular motions. Remove the cleanser using 4" x 4" moistened gauze pads or chosen material. Complete Procedure 5–1: Skin Analysis.			
3. Using 2" x 2" esthetic wipes or cotton rounds moistened with toner, remove any residue.			
4. Using a disposable spatula or brush apply the enzyme mask to the back area.			
5. Process the mask according to the manufacturer's instructions. (Remove sooner if client cannot tolerate the treatment or if the peel has processed prior to the recommended minimal end time.)			
6. Remove the mask using warm towels, 4" x 4" moistened esthetic wipes, or chosen material.			
7. Option: Perform extractions.			
8. Using 2" x 2" esthetic wipes or cotton rounds moistened with toner, remove any residue.			
9. Using a disposable spatula or brush apply a mask suitable for the client's skin type to the back area.			
10. Process the mask.			
11. Remove the mask using warm towels, 4" x 4" moistened esthetic wipes or chosen material.			
12. Apply moisturizer in circular motions and then sun protection.			
13. Remove your gloves and wash your hands.			
14. Discuss your observations and any recommendations with the client.			
15. Perform Procedure 7–2 and 8–9: Post-Service.			

PROCEDURE 13–3: PERFORM A LIGHT GLYCOLIC PEEL

Evaluate your practical skills.

CRITERIA	COMPETENT	NEEDS WORK	IMPROVEMENT PLAN
Procedure			
1. Complete Procedure 7–1: Pre-Service. Ensure the client is cleared for this service prior to proceeding.			
2. Cleanse and analyze the skin. Apply a cleanser suitable for the client's skin type with your gloved hands. Massage the cleanser in circular motions. Remove the cleanser using 4" x 4" moistened gauze pads or chosen material. Complete Procedure 5–1: Skin Analysis.			
3. Using 2" x 2" esthetic wipes or cotton rounds moistened with toner, remove any residue.			
4. Apply a protective ointment around the eyes, corners or the nose and on the lips.			
5. Apply protective eyewear to your client and then to yourself.			
6. Carefully analyze the client's skin with the magnifying lamp.			
7. Using a large tipped cotton swab, apply the peel beginning at the forehead and moving to the temples, then to the right and left cheeks, chin, upper lip, and nose.			
8. Process the peel according to the manufacturer's instructions (neutralize and remove sooner if client cannot tolerate the treatment or if the peel has processed prior to the recommended minimal end time). Endpoint goal: mild erythema.			
9. Using 2" x 2" esthetic wipes or chosen material, neutralize the peel in the same order as applied unless you need to spot neutralize other areas first due to the peel reaching its endpoint sooner.			
10. Remove the peel using damp 4" x 4" esthetic wipes or chosen material.			
11. Apply moisturizer and sun protection liberally.			
12. Remove your gloves and wash your hands.			
13. Discuss your observations and any recommendations with the client.			
14. Perform Procedure 7–2 and 8–9: Post-Service.			

PROCEDURE 13–4: PERFORM CRYSTAL-FEE MICRODERMABRASION (DIAMOND TIP)

Evaluate your practical skills.

CRITERIA	COMPETENT	NEEDS WORK	IMPROVEMENT PLAN
Procedure			
1. Complete Procedure 7–1: Pre-Service. Ensure the client is cleared for this service prior to proceeding.			
2. Cleanse and analyze the skin. Apply a cleanser suitable for the client's skin type with your gloved hands. Massage the cleanser in circular motions. Remove the cleanser using 4" x 4" moistened gauze pads or chosen material. Complete Procedure 5–1: Skin Analysis.			
3. Using 2" x 2" esthetic wipes or cotton rounds moistened with toner, remove any residue.			
4. Apply goggles to protect the eye area.			
5. Engage the crystal-free handpiece with the hose of the microdermabrasion machine. Test the intensity of the suction over your gloved hand and adjust accordingly.			
6. Begin at the forehead, then move to the temples, to the right and left cheeks, chin, upper lip, and nose.			
7. Use light, even pressure holding the skin taut between the thumb and the forefinger as you move from one section to the next.			
8. The number of passes should range between one and three depending on the thickness and sensitivity of the client's skin, the machine settings and, the point the erythema occurs. More sensitive clients and areas receive fewer passes.			
9. Passes typically proceed as follows: horizontal, vertical, then diagonal. Passes can be performed independently over the entire face and then proceed to the next direction until the treatment is completed. However, cross-hatching with two passes consisting of a horizontal then vertical action is used most frequently.			
10. For smaller areas, such as the upper lip and nose, change the diamond tip size that best fits the area being treated.			
11. Using 2" x 2" esthetic wipes or cotton rounds moistened with toner, remove any residue.			
12. Apply moisturizer and sun protection.			
13. Remove your gloves and wash your hands.			
14. Discuss your observations and any recommendations with the client.			
15. Perform Procedure 7–2 and 8–9: Post-Service.			